# HANDBOOK OF PSYCHIATRIC DRUGS

D1125253

# HANDBOOK OF PSYCHIATRIC DRUGS

**Jeffrey A. Lieberman**

*Professor and Chair*
*Department of Psychiatry*
*Columbia University, College of Physicians and*
*Surgeons, and Director, New York State Psychiatric*
*Institute, New York, USA*

**Allan Tasman**

*Professor and Chair*
*Department of Psychiatry and Behavioral Sciences*
*University of Louisville School of Medicine, Louisville,*
*Kentucky, USA*

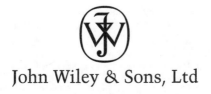

John Wiley & Sons, Ltd

*Other Wiley Editorial Offices*

John Wiley & Sons Inc., 111 River Street, Hoboken, NJ 07030, USA

Jossey-Bass, 989 Market Street, San Francisco, CA 94103-1741, USA

Wiley-VCH Verlag GmbH, Boschstr. 12, D-69469 Weinheim, Germany

John Wiley & Sons Australia Ltd, 42 McDougall Street, Milton, Queensland 4064,
Australia

John Wiley & Sons (Asia) Pte Ltd, 2 Clementi Loop #02-01, Jin Xing Distripark,
Singapore 129809

John Wiley & Sons Canada Ltd, 22 Worcester Road, Etobicoke, Ontario, Canada
M9W 1L1

Wiley also publishes its books in a variety of electronic formats. Some content that
appears in print may not be available in electronic books.

*Library of Congress Cataloging in Publication Data*

Lieberman, Jeffrey A., 1948–
    Handbook of psychiatric drugs / Jeffrey A. Lieberman, Allan Tasman.
      p.  cm.
    Includes bibliographical references and index.
    ISBN-13: 978-0-470-02821-6 (pbk. : alk. paper)
    ISBN-10: 0-470-02821-1 (pbk. : alk. paper)
    1. Psychotropic drugs—Handbooks, manuals, etc.  2. Psychopharmacology—
Handbooks, manuals, etc.  I. Tasman, Allan, 1947–  II. Title.
    RM315.L54 2006
    615′.788—dc22
                                2006004739

*British Library Cataloguing in Publication Data*

A catalogue record for this book is available from the British Library

ISBN-13 978-0-470-02821-6
ISBN-10 0-470-02821-1

Typeset in 9.5/11.5pt Times by Integra Software Services Pvt. Ltd, Pondicherry, India
Printed and bound in Great Britain by Clays Ltd, Bungay, Suffolk NR35 1ED
This book is printed on acid-free paper responsibly manufactured from sustainable
forestry in which at least two trees are planted for each one used for paper
production.

To our patients for their courage and for their assistance in the search for treatments for mental illness.

To my family in gratitude for their love, support and patience. *Jeffrey Lieberman*

With love and thanks to my family, and especially my father Goodman Tasman, for your inspiration and support. *Allan Tasman*

# CONTENTS

# PREFACE

There is little question that this is the most exciting time in history to be involved in the treatment of patients with psychiatric disorders. The explosive growth in our knowledge base in all areas of the field, particularly in neuroscience, has revolutionized both our understanding of the nature of psychiatric illnesses and our ability to provide effective treatments. As molecular genetics and pharmacology, neurochemistry, and new drug discovery techniques continue to advance, physicians are faced with the need to assimilate an ever-changing body of knowledge. In particular, the change in pharmacotherapy for psychiatric illnesses continues at a dizzying pace.

We have been very gratified by the extremely positive international response to our major textbook, *Psychiatry, Second Edition* (Tasman, A, Kay, J, Lieberman, JA, Wiley, 2003). We believe, however, that busy clinicians need a quick reference guide to the most up-to-date information on prescribing medications for psychiatric illnesses. This book, the *Handbook of Psychiatric Drugs*, is based on the outstanding chapters on pharmacotherapy in *Psychiatry, Second Edition*. The material has been condensed, updated to just months before publication, and organized by specific classes of medications. To enhance the daily utility of this handbook, we chose a format that emphasized ease of use, and ensured that each chapter follows a specific template of topics, including the pharmacology, mechanism of action and pharmacokinetics, indications and methods of prescribing, side effects and drug interactions, and descriptions of each specific drug within the class. We have aimed to include prescription medications in common use anywhere in the world. Further, each chapter was then reviewed by highly respected psychiatrists with pharmacotherapy expertise in that particular class of medication.

We feel confident that you will find this book to be one of your most useful sources of information regarding your daily clinical practice.

Jeffrey A. Lieberman, M.D.
New York, NY

Allan Tasman, M.D.
Louisville, KY

# ACKNOWLEDGEMENTS

We would like to gratefully acknowledge the authors of those chapters in *Psychiatry Second Edition* from which material in this book was adapted.

| | |
|---|---|
| Anri Aoba | Antipsychotic Drugs |
| Robert J. Boland | Antidepressants |
| W. Wolfgang Fleischhacker | Antipsychotic Drugs |
| Marlene P. Freeman | Mood Stabilizers |
| Alan J. Gelenberg | Mood Stabilizers |
| Laurence L. Greenhill | Stimulants |
| Jeffrey Halperin | Stimulants |
| Martin B. Keller | Antidepressants |
| Rachel E. Maddux | Anxiolytic Drugs |
| John March | Stimulants |
| Stephen R. Marder | Antipsychotic Drugs |
| John Misiaszek | Mood Stabilizers |
| Seiya Miyamoto | Antipsychotic Drugs |
| Scott E. Moseman | Mood Stabilizers |
| Mark H. Rapaport | Anxiolytic Drugs |
| Lon S. Schneider | Cognitive Enhancers and Treatments for Alzheimer's Disease |
| Richard I. Shader | Sedative–Hypnotic Agents |
| Erin Shockey | Stimulants |
| Douglas A. Songer | Sedative–Hypnotic Agents |
| Pierre N. Tariot | Cognitive Enhancers and Treatments for Alzheimer's Disease |

We also acknowledge Jeffrey Selzer, author of the chapter 'Drugs for Treating Substance Abuse in Psychiatric Drugs'.

We would also like to thank our colleagues from the College of Physicians and Surgeons of Columbia University, New York, who contributed to the final editing process:

D.P. Devanand
Laurence Greenhill
David J. Hellerstein
Edward V. Nunes
Lazlo Papp
David J. Printz
Zafar Sharif

# DISCLAIMER

# 1

# ANTIPSYCHOTIC DRUGS

## INTRODUCTION

Information about antipsychotic drugs and developments in the treatment of psychosis is rapidly expanding. The advent of newer second-generation antipsychotics in the wake of clozapine represents the first significant advances in the pharmacologic treatment of schizophrenia and related psychotic disorders, and second-generation antipsychotics have become first-choice agents for acute and maintenance therapy for these illnesses.

There is growing evidence that most of the new medications can offer advantages over conventional neuroleptics; these include fewer extrapyramidal symptoms, lower risk of tardive dyskinesia, reduced cognitive impairment, and possible improvement in negative symptoms. Treatment successes have contributed to the increased use of newer antipsychotic agents and have also allowed psychiatrists to expand clinical expectations. In addition, these second-generation drugs are being used increasingly for various conditions beyond schizophrenia, as happened with the conventional antipsychotics.

## PHARMACOLOGY

The first-generation antipsychotic agents are equally effective in the treatment of psychotic symptoms of schizophrenia, although they vary in potency and their propensity to induce various side effects. All have a high affinity for dopamine

*Handbook of Psychiatric Drugs*   Jeffrey A. Lieberman and Allan Tasman
© 2006 John Wiley & Sons, Ltd

$D_2$ receptors. In addition, all produce extra-pyramidal symptoms (EPS), including parkinsonism, dystonia, akathisia, are associated with a substantial risk of tardive dyskinesia (TD), and increase serum prolactin concentration in the usual clinical dose range. First-generation agents are usually classified into three groups: phenothiazines, butyrophenones (e.g., haloperidol), and others (e.g., thiothixene, molindone, and loxapine), based on their structure.

Second-generation antipsychotic drugs are characterized by the following criteria:

- few or no EPS; significant reduction in tardive dyskinesia liability compared to first-generation antipsychotics
- expanded spectrum of therapeutic efficacy
- less prolactin elevation

There is a continuum of typical and atypical effects in atypical drugs rather than several dichotomous groups.

## Chemistry

Antipsychotic drugs bind to numerous neurotransmitter receptor subtypes, including those of dopamine, norepinephrine, epinephrine, acetylcholine, serotonin, and histamine. They act to antagonize the endogenous ligands at these receptors. Both therapeutic and extrapyramidal side effects can be attributed to the antagonism of dopamine at $D_2$ receptors, with actions at the other neuroreceptors associated with various other side effects.

The typical antipsychotics have been described as being of high (e.g., haloperidol), low (e.g., chlorpromazine), and mid (e.g., loxapine) potency on the basis of their degree of affinity for $D_2$ receptors and their therapeutic dose range. Atypical antipsychotics are characterized by generally lower affinities for $D_2$ receptors and relatively greater affinities for serotonin (5-hydroxytryptamine) $5\text{-HT}_{2A}$ receptors in particular, but also for noradrenergic receptors ($\alpha_1$ and $\alpha_2$), muscarinic acetylcholine receptors, histamine, and other dopamine (DA) subtype receptors. Aripiprazole is currently the only antipsychotic that acts as a partial agonist at $D_2$ and $5\text{-HT}_{1A}$ receptors as well as an antagonist at the $5\text{-HT}_{2A}$ and $D_2$ receptors, and these properties are believed to account for its therapeutic effects. It has no appreciable activity at muscarinic receptors and modest affinity for alpha-1 adrenergic and histamine $H_1$ receptors.

## Mechanism of Action

The therapeutic actions of antipsychotic drugs are generally attributed to antagonism of DA receptors, particularly the $D_2$ subtype. Atypical antipsychotics, with their lower $D_2$ receptor affinities and broader spectrum of pharmacologic properties, also antagonize $5\text{-}HT_{2A}$ receptors, giving possible therapeutic advantages and a superior motor side effect profile. At this point it is unclear what clinical effects $5\text{-}HT_{2A}$ antagonism confers, other than mitigating the adverse effect of striatal $D_2$ antagonism, and propensity to cause EPS. The low EPS liability of aripiprazole is at least in part related to its partial agonist activity at the $D_2$ receptor. Its $D_2$ antagonist activity is broadly comparable with that of haloperidol and chlorpromazine, but it clearly has weaker cataleptogenic activity. Furthermore, chronic treatment with aripiprazole is associated with much less upregulation of striatal $D_2$ receptors compared with haloperidol.

What has been established is that as a consequence of their different pharmacologic profile, the atypical drugs have a much wider separation of the dose-response curves of therapeutic antipsychotic action and extrapyramidal side effects.

## Pharmacokinetics

Antipsychotic agents are rapidly absorbed from the gastrointestinal tract and undergo extensive first pass metabolism. They are highly lipophilic, which results in ready transport across the blood-brain barrier. Antipsychotics are metabolized by the cytochrome P450 enzyme system. The isozyme systems predominantly involved are CYP2D6, CYP1A2, CYP3A4, and CYP2C19, and medications that inhibit or compete for these substrates can increase antipsychotic blood levels. After undergoing various degrees of metabolism, antipsychotic drugs and their metabolites are glucuronidated in the liver and excreted by the kidney in the urine or in feces.

The average plasma half-life of the antipsychotics as a family is approximately 20 to 24 hours, allowing for once-daily dosing. Aripiprazole and its active metabolite dehydro-aripiprazole have exceptionally long half-lives of 75 and 94 hours respectively and steady state concentrations are achieved after 14 days. Some drugs have shorter half-lives (e.g., quetiapine: 6 to 12 hours; ziprasidone: 4 to 10 hours), which suggests twice-daily administration. However, with repeated dosing the pharmacodynamic effects may extend beyond the period suggested by pharmacokinetic parameters, allowing the consolidation of dosing to once daily.

Among the second-generation antipsychotics, olanzapine (5–10 mg initial dose) and ziprasidone (10–20 mg initial dose) are available in a parenteral form for acute use in agitated patients, giving the benefits of a more rapid onset of action and the ability to bypass the extensive first-pass metabolism that these agents undergo.

Several of the antipsychotic drugs (three in the United States: haloperidol and fluphenazine decanoate, and Risperidone – Risperdal Consta) are available in long-acting injectable preparations for intramuscular administration. This allows for less fluctuation in plasma level compared to oral formulations, bypasses first-pass metabolism, and can improve patient compliance.

Recommended dosages for second-generation antipsychotic agents are shown in Table 1-1.

## INDICATIONS FOR USE OF ANTIPSYCHOTIC DRUGS

Antipsychotic agents are effective for treating nearly every medical and psychiatric condition where psychotic symptoms or aggression are present. They are currently used routinely in the management of psychosis and/or agitation associated with:

- Schizophrenia and Schizoaffective Disorder
- Acute manic and mixed episodes of bipolar disorder
- Major depression with psychosis
- Delusional disorder
- Delirium
- Dementia
- Mental retardation
- Developmental disorders (e.g., Autism)
- Huntington's disease
- Tourette's syndrome
- Substance-induced psychoses (psychostimulants, phencyclidine, levodopa, steroids)

**TABLE 1-1.** Antipsychotic Drugs, Doses, Forms, and Costs

| DRUG CLASS | THERAPEUTIC DOSE RANGE: USUAL ORAL DAILY DOSE (mg/d) | THERAPEUTIC EQUIVALENT ORAL DOSE (mg/d) | FORMS | HALF-LIFE (h) |
|---|---|---|---|---|
| **First-generation antipsychotics** | | | | |
| Perphenazine | 8–64 | 10 | Tablets (2, 4, 8, 16 mg)<br>Concentrate (16 mg/5 ml)<br>Injectable solution (5 mg/ml) | 9 |
| Chlorpromazine | 200–1,000 | 100 | Tablets (10, 25, 50, 100, 200 mg)<br>Concentrate (30, 100 mg/ml)<br>Gel Caps (30 mg)<br>Spansules (30, 75, 150 mg)<br>Injectable solution (25 mg/ml)<br>Rectal suppositories (25 mg) | 23–37 |
| Haloperidol | 2–20 | 2 | Tablets (0.5, 1, 2, 5, 10, 20 mg)<br>Concentrate (2 mg/ml)<br>Injectable solution (5 mg/ml) | 24 |
| **Second-generation antipsychotics** | | | | |
| Risperidone | 2–8 | 1–2 | Tablets (0.25, 0.5, 1, 2, 3, 4 mg)<br>Concentrate (1 mg/ml)<br>M-tabs (0.5, 1, 2 mg) rapidly disintegrating tablets<br>Risperdal Consta long-acting injectable (25, 37.5, 50 mg) q 2 wk | Parent 3<br>Metabolite 24 |

■ **TABLE 1-1.** (Continued)

| DRUG CLASS | THERAPEUTIC DOSE RANGE: USUAL ORAL DAILY DOSE (mg/d) | THERAPEUTIC EQUIVALENT ORAL DOSE (mg/d) | FORMS | HALF-LIFE (h) |
|---|---|---|---|---|
| Ziprasidone | 80–200 | 20 | Capsules (20, 40, 60, 80 mg) Injectable solution 20 mg/ml | 4–10 |
| Clozapine | 25–600 | 50 | Tablets (25, 100 mg) | 8–12 |
| Olanzapine | 5–30 | 2.5–5 | Tablets (2.5, 5, 7.5, 10, 15, 20 mg) Zydis (5, 10, 15, 20 mg) rapidly disintegrating tablets Injectable solution 5 mg/ml | 27 |
| Quetiapine | 150–800 | 50–100 | Tablets (25, 50, 100, 200, 300, 400 mg) | 7 |
| Aripiprazole | 10–30 | 5–10 | Tablets (5, 10, 15, 20, 30 mg) Oral solution 1 mg/ml | 75–96 |
| **Long-acting preparations** | | | | |
| Fluphenazine decanoate | 12.5–50 q 2–4 wk | 12.5–50 | Injectable solution (25 mg/ml) | 2–3 wk |
| Haloperidol decanoate | 50–300 q 3–4 wk | 50–300 | Injectable solution (100 mg/ml) | 3 wk |
| Risperdal Consta | 25–50 mg q 2 wk | 25, 37.5, 50 mg | Microspheres in fixed dose vials; 2 ml | 3–6 days |

Adapted and reprinted from Lieberman JA and Mendelowitz AJ (2000). Antipsychotic Drugs, Doses, Forms, and Costs. In *Psychiatric Drugs*, Lieberman JA and Tasman A (eds.) WB Saunders, pp. 1–43. © 2000, with permission from Elsevier.

The development of second-generation antipsychotics has been a major clinical advance for the treatment of schizophrenia. At present, these drugs are used as the first-line treatment for schizophrenia, and are being used increasingly for various conditions beyond schizophrenia. The low incidence of EPS and TD associated with second-generation agents is highly beneficial in several neuropsychiatric conditions.

## DRUG SELECTION AND INITIATION OF TREATMENT

### Drug Selection for the Treatment of Schizophrenia

In choosing an antipsychotic agent for the treatment of an episode of schizophrenia, the clinician should be guided by the patient's history. The following tests should be performed:

- a complete physical examination including weight
- a review of symptoms
- routine blood chemistry including fasting blood glucose and lipid profile
- complete blood cell count
- electrocardiogram

Once any medical or neurologic causes of the symptoms have been ruled out, the clinician should consider the following questions:

- Is this a psychotic episode consistent with schizophrenia?
- Have affective syndromes such as mania and depression with psychotic features been ruled out?
- Is this the patient's first episode?
- Is there a history of prior antipsychotic treatment response?
- How well was the antipsychotic tolerated?
- Were there prominent side effects?
- Did the patient ever previously have EPS or TD?
- Does the patient have a history of neuroleptic malignant syndrome?
- What symptoms (positive or negative) are predominant in the episode?

- Is there a history of non-compliance, and, if so, has the patient had a trial of depot preparations?
- If there have been antipsychotic trials that have failed, were the trials of an adequate dose and of an adequate duration?
- Does the patient meet the criteria for treatment resistance?
- Does the patient have a history of cardiac conduction delay?
- Does the patient have any prior history of blood dyscrasias?
- Does the patient have normal hepatic and renal functions?
- Is the patient medically debilitated?

**TREATMENT INITIATION AND DOSE TITRATION**
Once the questions above are answered, the clinician should select an antipsychotic medication and initiate the treatment trial. The algorithm from the practice guidelines for schizophrenia developed by the American Psychiatric Association may be useful for drug selection (Figure 1-1).

Selection of an agent in emergency settings for the management of the gross agitation, excitement, and violent behavior associated with psychosis might be based on clinical symptoms, differences in efficacy or side effects of candidate drugs, or, more pragmatically, the formulation of a drug as it affects route of administration, onset, and duration.

There is now a considerable amount of clinical experience with atypical antipsychotics in acute emergency situations, and they have come to replace first-generation antipsychotics as the agents of choice when treatment is initiated. Olanzapine and ziprasidone are available in short-acting formulations for intramuscular administration; risperidone and aripiprazole are available as oral solutions; and olanzapine and risperidone are available as rapidly disintegrating oral tablets. These various formulations provide tremendous flexibility to the clinician in choosing the optimal medication and method of administration based on clinical considerations.

The use of oral second-generation antipsychotics and benzodiazepines in combination is the most common medication strategy in psychiatric emergency settings. It is best to avoid combining antipsychotics in favor of sequential trials of monotherapy with different antipsychotics. Because most patients with schizophrenia will require long-term treatment with antipsychotics it is imperative that, in addition to short-term treatment goals of control of behavioral dysregulation

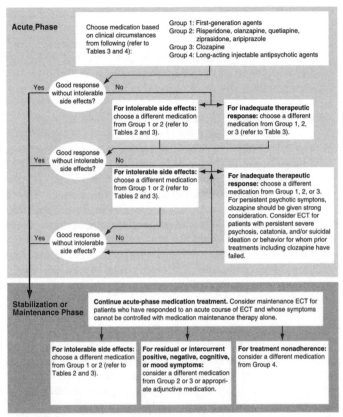

**FIGURE 1-1.** Somatic Treatment of Schizophrenia. Also refer to Table 1-1 and the following: First episode–Group(G) 2; Persistent suicidal ideation or behavior–G3; Persistent hostility and aggressive behavior–G3; Tardive dyskinesia–G2 all group 2 drugs may not be equal in their lower or no tardive dyskinesia liability and G3; History of sensitivity to extrapyramidal side effects–G2 except higher doses of risperidone; History of sensitivity to prolactin elevation–G2 except risperidone; History of sensitivity to weight gain, hyperglycemia, or hyperlipidemia–G2 ziprasidone or aripiprazole; Repeated nonadherence to pharmacological treatment–G4 (taken from the Practice Guidelines for the Treatment of Patients with Bipolar Disorder, Second Edition from the American Psychiatric Association Practice Guidelines for the Treatment of Psychiatric Disorders Compendium, Copyright 2004).

and psychotic symptom resolution, clinicians consider long-term side effect profiles of the available treatment options with the goal of minimizing long-term side effect burden. Ziprasidone and aripiprazole may be specifically indicated in patients who are intolerant of the side effects that can occur in greater frequency with some of the second-generation drugs, such as weight gain and alterations in glucose and lipid metabolism, as they do not produce these effects to any significant degree.

One can safely escalate the dose of second-generation antipsychotics more rapidly than is usual in outpatient settings to achieve target doses typically utilized for the treatment of schizophrenia. Once behavioral control is achieved, benzodiazepines should be discontinued and the patient should be maintained on the atypical antipsychotic alone. The dose recommendations for second-generation antipsychotic drugs are summarized in Table 1-2.

The anti-aggressive characteristics of clozapine are well established in chronically psychotic patients; however clozapine initiation is contraindicated in the psychiatric emergency setting because of its serious potential side effects, including seizures and agranulocytosis.

On the rare occasion that a physician elects to use a first-generation antipsychotic during the first few days of treatment, "rapid neuroleptization" should be avoided as there is no evidence for increased efficacy and risk of side effects is greater at higher doses. If a low-potency agent is chosen, the recommendation is to begin with a low dose such as chlorpromazine, 50 mg twice a day, and to titrate slowly so that the difficulties associated with orthostatic hypotension can be reduced. If a high-potency agent such as haloperidol is chosen, the recommendation is also to begin a course of prophylactic antiparkinsonism medication such as benztropine, 1 mg twice a day, to decrease the incidence of EPS side effects. The initial dose of antipsychotic should be titrated to between 5 and 10 haloperidol equivalents or 200 to 400 chlorpromazine equivalents. At this time, the only groups of patients in which the first-generation antipsychotics are clearly preferable are those who have a history of good response to these agents with minimal side effects.

After initiating treatment and titrating to a standard dose of antipsychotic, the clinician, patient, and family must wait for the antipsychotic to take effect. Because patients are acutely

■ **TABLE 1-2.** Recommended Dosages for Second-Generation Antipsychotic Agents

| | HALF-LIFE (hr) (MEAN) | STARTING DOSE (TOTAL mg/day) | AVERAGE DOSE RANGE (mg/day) | | AVERAGE MAINTENANCE DOSE (mg/day) | ROUTES OF ADMINISTRATION |
|---|---|---|---|---|---|---|
| | | | FIRST EPISODE | RECURRENT EPISODE | | |
| Clozapine | 10–105 (16) | 25–50 | 150–300 | 400–600 | 400 | Oral |
| Risperidone | 3–24 (15) | 1–2 | 2–4 | 3–6 | 3–6 | Oral, depot |
| Olanzapine | 20–70 (30) | 5–10 | 10–20 | 15–30 | 10–20 | Oral, IM |
| Quetiapine | 4–10 (7) | 50–100 | 300–600 | 500–800 | 400–800 | Oral |
| Ziprasidone | 4–10 | 40–80 | 80–120 | 120–200 | 120–160 | Oral, IM |
| Zotepine | 12–30 (15) | 50–100 | 75–150 | 150–450 | 75–300 | Oral |
| Amisulpride | 8–20 (12) | 50–100 | 50–300 | 400–800 | 400–800 | Oral |
| Aripiprazole | (75–96) | 10–15 | 10–30 | 15–30 | 15–30 | Oral |

*Source:* Adapted from McEvoy JP, Scheifler PL, Frances A (1999) The expert consensus guideline series: Treatment of schizophrenia. *J Clin Psychiatr* 60, 1–80; Burns MJ (2001) The pharmacology and toxicology of atypical antipsychotic agents. *J Clin Toxicol* 39, 1–14; Worrel JA, Marken PA, Beckman SE, et al. (2000) Atypical antipsychotic agents: A critical review. *Am J Health Syst Pharm* 57, 238–255.

ill, there is often a tremendous temptation and external pressure to increase the dose of the antipsychotic in the hope that the patient's condition will improve more rapidly. Despite this hope, there is little, if any, clinical evidence that a higher dose of antipsychotic is in any way advantageous; in fact, it will only increase the likelihood of side effects. During this difficult time it may be necessary to add sedating medications such as short-acting benzodiazepines (e.g., lorazepam) to help the patient maintain control until the antipsychotic has started to work.

## TREATMENT EVALUATION AND DRUG SWITCHING

If the first-episode patient has failed to respond to a 6-week trial of an antipsychotic, the clinician should evaluate possible non-compliance with medication, the likelihood of a partial response or a complete nonresponse to treatment. If there was no response, a change to a second antipsychotic from a new family is recommended. If one of the newer agents was not the clinician's first choice, it should be used at this point in the decision tree.

If a patient has already discontinued use of a medication, then the new treatment is selected and initiated as described above. However, if the patient is undergoing maintenance drug treatment and drugs are to be electively switched in the hope of achieving a better therapeutic response or alleviating drug side effects, then the goal is to switch medications without destabilizing the patient.

Medication changes should be performed by a concurrent slow tapering of the initial antipsychotic while the second antipsychotic is being slowly titrated. The specific rate of cross-titration depends on the dose of the old medication and the relative stability of the patient. In general, the higher the dose and the more unstable the patient, the longer and more gradual the cross-titration schedule. Although this varies, a rule of thumb is to cross-titrate by yoked increments and decrements of 25% every 2 to 5 days. Adjunctive medications should be adjusted or tapered accordingly.

If the patient is judged to be a partial responder to the antipsychotic trial, then the clinician may consider the addition of an agent for augmentation. At this point, it is again important for the clinician to re-evaluate the presence of affective symptoms. If there is significant depressive symtomatology in the clinical presentation, then the addition of an antidepressant may be warranted. If the presence of mood symptoms is consistent with a manic episode, the addition of a mood stabilizer such as lithium as an augmentation strategy may be clinically useful.

***Treatment During the Resolving Phase*** If a particular antipsychotic medication has improved the acute symptoms it should be continued at the same dose for the next six months before a lower maintenance dose is considered for continued treatment. Rapid dose reduction or discontinuation of the medications during the resolving phase may result in relatively rapid relapse. It is essential to continue to assess side effects present in the acute phase and modify treatment to minimize their negative impact, and to re-evaluate the necessity of any adjunctive therapies used in the acute phase.

If the decision has been made to switch to a long-acting depot antipsychotic agent, this can often be achieved during this phase. This is also a good time to educate the patient and family regarding the course and outcome of schizophrenia, as well as factors that influence the outcome such as drug compliance.

## MAINTENANCE TREATMENT

The goals of treatment during the stable or maintenance phase are to maintain symptom remission, to prevent psychotic relapse, to implement a plan for rehabilitation, and to improve the patient's quality of life.

Current guidelines recommend that first-episode patients should be treated for one to two years; however, 75% of patients will experience relapses after their treatment is discontinued. Patients who have had multiple episodes should receive at least five years of maintenance therapy. Patients with severe or dangerous episodes should probably be treated indefinitely.

Gradual dose reduction to identify the minimum effective dose for the patient can be attempted in this phase, although relapse rates are excessively high when doses are reduced to about 10% of the acute dose.

Antipsychotics have been proven to be effective in reducing the risk of psychotic relapse in maintenance therapy for schizophrenia. In the stable phase of illness, antipsychotics can reduce the risk of relapse to less than 30% per year.

Without maintenance treatment, 60–70% of patients relapse within one year and almost 90% relapse within two years. These results indicate that antipsychotic medications are effective in preventing relapse in most stabilized patients. There is also strong evidence that patients who relapsed while on antipsychotic medications had episodes that were less severe than patients not on antipsychotic drugs.

As atypical drugs have fewer EPS side effects, patients on these compounds may be less likely to be non-compliant with treatment and may thereby decrease their risk of relapse. It has also been suggested that in addition to fewer side effects, atypical drugs may have inherently greater prophylactic efficacy than typical drugs and therefore be better for patients with an increased risk of relapse.

## TREATING TREATMENT RESISTANCE

Treatment resistance is generally defined as a failure of two prior drug trials of 4–6 weeks duration. Although most definitions of treatment resistance focus on the persistence of positive symptoms, there is growing awareness of the problems of persistent negative symptoms and cognitive impairments, which may have an important impact on level of functioning, psychosocial integration, and quality of life.

Approximately 10 to 15% of patients with first-episode schizophrenia are resistant to drug treatment, and between 25% and 50% of long-term patients will have severe, persistent symptoms including psychosis.

Only clozapine has consistently demonstrated efficacy for psychotic symptoms in well-defined treatment refractory patients; the mechanism responsible for this therapeutic advantage remains uncertain. Serum levels of $350 \mu g/mL$ or greater have been associated with maximal likelihood of response. Depending on the type of residual symptom, augmentation strategies include adding another antipsychotic, anticonvulsants, benzodiazepines, and cholinergic agonists may prove useful.

Since the approval of clozapine, attention has shifted to a greater focus on the use of other second-generation antipsychotics for managing treatment resistance in schizophrenia. Both olanzapine (15–25 mg/day) and clozapine (200–600 mg/day) were shown to be similarly effective in reducing overall psychotic symptoms in treatment-resistant patients clinically eligible for treatment with clozapine. Some preliminary reports suggest that higher doses of olanzapine may be more effective; however, dosage issues of olanzapine have not yet been adequately addressed in more controlled conditions. There are also several recent reports of beneficial effects of quetiapine in treatment-resistant patients with schizophrenia.

Given the risk of agranulocytosis, the burden of side effects, and the requirement of white blood cell monitoring, the second-generation agents (risperidone, olanzapine, quetiapine, ziprasidone, and aripiprazole) should be tried in almost all patients before proceeding to clozapine. Many clinicians express the impression that certain patients do respond preferentially to a single agent of this class.

### SCHIZOAFFECTIVE DISORDER AND VIOLENT PATIENTS

Among the specific therapeutic effects claimed for atypical drugs is their ability to alleviate mood symptoms associated with the psychotic disorder. Although this has not been definitively proved, preliminary results indicate that mood symptoms may selectively abate with atypical drugs. This evidence suggests that patients with schizoaffective disorder, residual mood symptoms (e.g., postpsychotic depression), a history of, or current, suicidal behavior, and violent behavior may benefit most from treatment with an atypical drug as compared to a conventional antipsychotic agent.

### ADJUNCTIVE TREATMENTS

For patients who are unresponsive to antipsychotic agents, including clozapine, and for patients who are responsive but have substantial residual symptoms, the question is what further options exist. Adjunctive medications as indicated in the algorithm (other than electroconvulsive therapy) have been used extensively but without any empiric data to demonstrate their efficacy. These adjuncts include anticonvulsants, lithium, antidepressants, benzodiazepines, and cholinesterase inhibitors.

## Effects of Antipsychotic Agents on Symptoms of Schizophrenia

The clinical profile of second-generation antipsychotic agents on the symptoms of schizophrenia are summarized in Table 1-3.

■ **TABLE 1-3.** Clinical Profile of Second-Generation Antipsychotic Drug Efficacy

| DRUG | CLOZAPINE | RISPERIDONE | OLANZAPINE | QUETIAPINE | ZIPRASIDONE | SERTINDOLE | AMISULPRIDE | ARIPIPRAZOLE | ILOPERIDONE |
|---|---|---|---|---|---|---|---|---|---|
| **Clinical effect** | | | | | | | | | |
| Psychotic symptoms | +++ | +++ | +++ | ++ | ++ | +++ | +++ | +++ | +++ |
| Negative symptoms | + | + | + | + | + | ++ | ++ | ++ | ++ |
| Cognitive symptoms | ++ | ++ | ++ | + | ? | ? | ? | ++ | ? |
| Mood symptoms | +++ | ++ | +++ | +++ | ++ | ++ | ++ | ++ | ? |
| Refractory symptoms | +++ | ++ | ++ | ++ | ? | ? | ++ | ? | ? |

+ to +++, weakly to strongly active; ?, questionable to unknown activity.
*Source:* Adapted from Dawkins K, Lieberman JA, Lebowitz BD, et al. (1999) Antipsychotics: Past and future. National Institute of Mental Health Division of Services and Intervention Research Workshop (July 14, 1998). *Schizophr Bull* 25, 395–404, with permission from Oxford University Press.

***Positive Symptoms*** Antipsychotic agents have a specific effect on positive symptoms of schizophrenia including hallucinations, delusions, and thought disorder. Approximately 30% of patients with acutely exacerbated psychotic symptoms have little or no response to conventional antipsychotics, and up to 50% of patients have only a partial response to medication. Although the proportion of patients who improve and the magnitude of therapeutic effects vary greatly, second-generation antipsychotics appear to be at least as effective for psychotic symptoms as conventional drugs.

***Negative Symptoms*** Studies of the early course of illness have shown that about 70% of schizophrenics develop primary negative symptoms such as affective blunting, emotional withdrawal, poverty of speech, anhedonia, and apathy, before the onset of positive symptoms. Negative symptoms may represent core features of the illness, and may be associated with poor outcome and prolonged hospitalization for patients.

Negative symptoms can be divided into three components that are usually difficult to distinguish:

- primary or deficit – enduring negative symptoms
- primary – non-enduring negative symptoms
- secondary negative symptoms that may be associated with psychotic symptoms, EPS, depression, and environmental deprivation

Conventional antipsychotics are generally less effective against negative than positive symptoms of schizophrenia; thus, the efficacy of second-generation antipsychotics on negative symptoms compared with that of first-generation drugs has received much attention. Second-generation agents such as clozapine, olanzapine and risperidone demonstrate significantly greater efficacy than conventional agents in reducing negative symptoms.

However, there is a continuing debate as to whether these effects are related to a reduction in EPS or to a direct effect on primary negative symptoms. Moreover, the effect sizes of improvement on negative symptoms for second-generation agents are usually moderate to small in comparison with placebo or conventional agents. Path analyses have suggested that both risperidone and olanzapine exert direct effects on (primary) negative symptoms independent of differences in psychotic, depressive, or extrapyramidal symptoms. A collaborative working group concluded that second-generation drugs are superior in terms of the "totality" of negative symptoms, but their impact on specific components is still under investigation. This and other clinical questions will become clear as the new agents are tested in clinical trials.

***Cognitive Symptoms*** Cognitive impairment appears to be an integral characteristic of schizophrenia and may be evident in up to 60% of patients. Measurable deficits are prominent in tasks involving attention, verbal fluency, memory, and executive function. A wide range of cognitive deficits are usually present at the time of the first psychotic episode and remain relatively stable or only slowly progressive during the course of the illness, independent of psychotic symptoms. Cognitive deficits are particularly prominent in patients meeting criteria for the deficit syndrome and in patients with TD. They are more strongly related to social and vocational functioning than psychotic symptoms and may influence the quality of life of patients. Thus, targeting cognitive impairments appears to be a major focus of the treatment of schizophrenia.

Conventional neuroleptics produce small and inconsistent effects on cognitive functioning. In general, clozapine, risperidone, and olanzapine have demonstrated superior efficacy compared to first-generation antipsychotics on tests of verbal fluency, digit–symbol substitution, fine motor function, and executive function. Measures of learning and memory were least affected by second-generation agents. Because these tests all measure performance during a timed trial, enhanced performance with second-generation drugs could result, in part, from reduced parkinsonian side effects. Preliminary evidence suggests that risperidone may be more effective for visual and working memory than clozapine.

***Mood Symptoms and Suicidal Behavior*** Depressive symptoms frequently occur in the context of psychotic symptoms or intercurrently between psychotic episodes. Antidepressant medication used adjunctively to antipsychotic drugs is generally indicated and effective. Atypical antipsychotics have been reported to have selective benefits against mood symptoms in schizophrenia, both manic and depressive.

Suicidal behavior presents a particular problem in patients with schizophrenia. Clozapine is approved for use in suicidal patients with schizophrenia on the basis of results in the InterSePT study. This study found that clozapine treatment produced a lower rate of suicidal behavior than the comparison treatment of olanzapine in patients with active or histories of suicidal behavior.

## Drug Selection for the Treatment of Bipolar Disorder

Antipsychotic agents are effective in treating acute manic episodes; these agents are believed to possess antimanic qualities in addition to their antipsychotic properties. One benefit is their rapid onset compared to mood stabilizers; as a result, these agents are often used preferentially or combined until the mood stabilizer has reached its therapeutic effectiveness. All the second-generation antipsychotics (except clozapine) are now approved for the treatment of acute manic episode in the United States, as well as the acute treatment of mixed episodes (except clozapine and quetiapine). Olanzapine and aripiprazole are also approved for maintenance treatment.

A concern with the use of antipsychotics in this population is the potential for TD. As a result, it is recommended that atypical antipsychotics be used with this population when clinically indicated but that attempts be made to treat this population with mood-stabilizing agents by themselves if possible.

## Drug Selection for the Treatment of Major Depression With Psychotic Features

Clear psychotic symptoms, such as delusions or hallucinations, are observed in approximately 25% of patients with major depressive disorder. These symptoms often respond poorly to antidepressants when they are administered alone, and usually require the use of adjunctive antipsychotic agents.

Treatment can be initiated simultaneously, though many clinicians prefer to start the antipsychotic dose first and then add the antidepressant to the regimen. Though there are limited data on the adequate dose of antipsychotic for this group, most clinicians would recommend 5 to 10 haloperidol equivalents. This group of unipolar depressed patients may be at the highest risk of TD; thus the antipsychotic dosage should be tapered and then discontinued when the patient's psychotic symptoms remit.

## Drug Selection for the Treatment of Delusional Disorder

Delusional disorder differs from other psychotic disorders in terms of family history and age distribution. In addition, it has displayed a difference in treatment response; as a general rule, patients with delusional disorder do not respond well to antipsychotic agents. Some uncontrolled clinical data have suggested that these patients may do better with drugs from the diphenylbutylpiperidine class (e.g., pimozide). However, the majority of this group of patients are untreated and do not seek psychiatric help. There is only very limited experience with atypical drugs in this population.

## Drug Selection for the Treatment of Delirium

Antipsychotics are effective in treating the psychotic symptoms and agitation associated with deliria of various etiologies. In treating a delirium, high-potency agents are preferable to low-potency agents because low-potency agents usually have more anticholinergic properties and cardiovascular side effects, which can adversely affect a delirious patient. Antipsychotic drugs are commonly given parenterally when used for this indication, including by intravenous routes.

Risperidone is also relatively free from anticholinergic side effects and has a favorable side-effect profile in relation to the production of EPS. The newer agents olanzapine and quetiapine are now being utilized for these conditions. The parenteral forms of the atypical drugs should be particularly useful for this indication.

## Drug Selection for the Treatment of Psychosis and Agitation Associated with Dementia

Antipsychotics are effective in treating the psychotic symptoms that are often associated with dementias. Additionally, they have been demonstrated to have anti-aggressive and calming effects against dysregulated behavior and affect. Although many patients with dementia have agitation and behavioral disturbances that clearly require the use of antipsychotic drugs, these drugs should be used judiciously.

The atypical drugs offer several potential advantages over typical drugs in treating dementia. They produce fewer EPS and less TD, side effects to which elderly patients are highly susceptible. They also may have broader efficacy against the constellation of pathologic symptoms and behaviors (e.g., mood symptoms, hostility) that occur in dementia. To date, extensive placebo-controlled trials have been conducted with risperidone, olanzapine and aripiprazole. Other atypical drugs must be systematically evaluated to determine their efficacy for this disorder and to determine how well their antiadrenergic and anticholinergic properties are tolerated.

Elderly patients with dementia who are treated with an antipsychotic agent are at increased risk of death. Analyses of clinical trials with a modal duration of 10 weeks suggest that the excess risk is 1.6–1.7 compared with placebo. Most of the deaths appear to be due to cardiovascular events (including heart failure and sudden death) or infection. Because these events have been associated with antipsychotics regardless of their chemical structure, this is probably a class effect associated with their pharmacological activity and the risk applies also to both atypical and older antipsychotics and to drugs that were not included in these trials. The FDA has reminded prescribers that these agents are not approved for the treatment of dementia in older people.

## Drug Selection for the Treatment of Mental Retardation and Developmental Disorders

Patients with mental retardation are another patient population with psychotic symptoms and behavioral disturbances about whom there has been controversy. As with patients with dementia, a number of these patients have documented psychosis, and for these patients the use of antipsychotics is clearly indicated. There are other patients, however, whose primary symptoms are those of behavioral dyscontrol. In this group it is possible that the risks of antipsychotics may outweigh their benefits, especially in long-term treatment. Again, atypical drugs may be advantageous because of their lower EPS and TD liabilities, to which these patients are highly susceptible.

## Drug Selection for Huntington's Disease and Tourette's Disorder

Antipsychotics have been shown to be effective in the management of Huntington's disease and Tourette's disorder. In Huntington's, various antipsychotics have been used to help control the agitation and chorea as well as the psychotic symptoms associated with the disorder. In Tourette's disorder, the antipsychotics used most extensively to manage patients' vocalizations and tics include haloperidol and pimozide. Most recently, risperidone has shown promise in this patient population. Beyond risperidone, there is little experience with atypical drugs in these disorders. The exception to this is clozapine, which was found to have little therapeutic benefit in either condition.

On the basis of this evidence, the typical drugs might be the preferred therapeutic option in these disorders; nonstriatal weak $D_2$ agents would be less likely to be effective.

## Substance-induced Psychoses

### PSYCHOSTIMULANT- AND PHENCYCLIDINE-INDUCED PSYCOSES

Substance intoxication resulting in psychotic symptoms may be treated effectively with antipsychotic drugs. This is particularly the case with intoxication from psychostimulants such as amphetamine, methamphetamine, and cocaine and from phencyclidine. Previously the clinical approach was not to use typical neuroleptics for fear of exacerbating the patient's condition with side effects but, rather, to employ benzodiazepines and a calm low-stimulus environment, unless the condition persisted for days or well beyond the period of the toxin's elimination. With the availability of the atypical drugs and their ability to alter the effects of NMDA receptor antagonists as well as psychostimulants, the use of these agents should be evaluated. At present, however, only limited data on their efficacy in these conditions are available.

### LEVODOPA-INDUCED AND STEROID-INDUCED PSYCHOSIS

Antipsychotics are an integral part of the treatment of medication-induced psychotic syndromes. The psychosis induced by levodopa in the treatment of Parkinson's disease presents unique clinical dilemmas. Treatment of the symptoms with first-generation antipsychotic agents will by definition worsen the Parkinson's symptoms. The clinician is often caught between attempts to reduce the patient's severe paranoid state and attempts to keep the patient from becoming more immobile from worsening rigidity and akinesia. Recently, case reports utilizing clozapine and risperidone in this population have shown encouraging results.

Steroid-induced psychotic symptoms have proved to be somewhat more complicated: psychotic symptoms may be prolonged, requiring the use of antipsychotics, and at the same time, despite the emergence of psychosis, some patients may still require steroid treatment for their medical condition. There have been a few case reports in which patients known to become psychotic during a steroid course were pretreated with antipsychotics or with a mood stabilizer, with good results.

## ADVERSE EFFECTS OF ANTIPSYCHOTICS

Antipsychotics as a group have a wide range of potential side effects corresponding to their pharmacologic properties. Atypical and typical drugs vary markedly in their side-effect profiles; clozapine has the most complicated and potentially serious side effects. The side effects for representative high-, mid-, and low-potency typical drugs and individual atypical drugs are shown in Table 1-4.

■ TABLE 1-4. Side-Effect Profile of Second-Generation Antipsychotic Drugs

| DRUG Side effect | CONVENTIONAL AGENTS | CLOZAPINE | RISPERIDONE | OLANZAPINE | QUETIAPINE | ZIPRASIDONE | SERTINDOLE | AMISULPRIDE | ARIPIPRAZOLE | ILOPERIDONE |
|---|---|---|---|---|---|---|---|---|---|---|
| EPS[a] | +++ | 0 | ++ | + | 0 | + | 0 | ++ | + | + |
| TD | +++ | 0 | ++ | + | 0 | + | 0 to + | + | + | + |
| NMS | ++ | + | + | + | ? | + | + | + | ? | ? |
| Prolactin elevation | +++ | 0 | +++ | 0 to + | 0 | 0 to + | 0 to + | ++ | 0 | 0 to + |
| Weight gain | + to ++ | +++ | + | +++ | + | 0 | + | + | 0 | ? |
| Prolonged QT[a] | + to +++ | 0 | + | 0 | + | ++ | +++ | + | 0 | 0 |
| Hypotension[a] | + to ++ | +++ | + | ++ | ++ | + | + | 0 | + | + |
| Sinus tachycardia[a] | + to +++ | +++ | + | ++ | ++ | + | + | 0 | 0 | + |
| Anticholinergic effects[a] | + to +++ | +++ | 0 | ++ | + | 0 | 0 | 0 | 0 | 0 |
| Hepatic transaminitis | + to ++ | ++ | + | ++ | + | + | + | + | 0 | + |
| Agranulo-cytosis | 0 to + | ++ | 0 | 0 | 0 | 0 | 0 | 0 | 0 | 0 |
| Sedation | + to +++ | +++ | + | ++ | +++ | + | + | + | + | + |
| Seizures[a] | 0 to + | +++ | 0 | 0 to + | 0 to + | 0 to + | 0 to + | 0 to + | 0 to + | 0 to + |

EPS, extrapyramidal side effects; TD, tardive dyskinesia; NMS, neuroleptic malignant syndrome.
+ to +++, active to strongly active; 0, minimal to none; ?, questionable to unknown activity.
[a] Dose dependent.

Adapted and modified with permission from Dawkins K, Lieberman JA, Lebowitz BD, et al. (1999) Antipsychotics: Past and future. National Institute of Mental Health Division of Services and Intervention Research Workshop (July 14, 1998). *Schizophr Bull* 25, 395–404; Burns MJ (2001) The pharmacology and toxicology of atypical antipsychotic agents. *J Clin Toxicol* 39, 1–14.

## Acute Extrapyramidal Side Effects (Dystonia, Parkinsonism, Akathisia)

Antipsychotic-induced EPS occur both acutely and after chronic treatment. All antipsychotic medications are capable of producing EPS. In general, first-generation antipsychotics are more likely to cause EPS than second-generation antipsychotics when the drugs are used at usual therapeutic doses. Among second-generation drugs, clozapine and quetiapine have been shown to carry minimal to no risk for EPS within the therapeutic dosage range. Risperidone can produce dose-related EPS ($\geq 6\,mg/day$). With the exception of akathisia, the incidence of EPS with olanzapine, aripiprazole, and ziprasidone is not appreciably different from that with placebo. The relative liability of the individual second-generation agents to produce EPS will become apparent only when they have been directly compared with each other in prospective clinical trials.

Commonly occurring acute EPS include akathisia, dystonia, and parkinsonism, with each having a characteristic time of onset. This group of acute EPS develops relatively soon after the initiation of antipsychotic medications and remits soon after the drugs are discontinued. These movement disorders are dose-dependent and reversible.

Dystonias tend to be sudden in onset, the most dramatic form of acute EPS, and extremely distressing to patients. They present as sustained muscle contraction with contorting, twisting, or abnormal postures affecting mainly the musculature of the head and neck but sometimes the trunk and lower extremities. Dystonic reactions usually occur within the first few days of therapy. Laryngeal dystonias are the most serious, and are potentially fatal. Risk factors for acute dystonias include a history of prior dystonias, young age, male gender, use of high-potency neuroleptic agents such as haloperidol or fluphenazine, high dose of medication, and parenteral administration.

Medication-induced parkinsonism is characterized by the symptoms of idiopathic parkinsonism, including rigidity, tremor, akinesia, and bradykinesia. Risk factors include older age, higher dose, a history of parkinsonism, and underlying damage in the basal ganglia.

Patients with akinesia or bradykinesia suffer from slow movement, apathy, and with difficulty with spontaneity of speech and initiating movement. These symptoms need to be distinguished from negative symptoms of schizophrenia, depressive symptoms, and catatonia.

Akathisia, the most common EPS of conventional antipsychotics agents, is characterized by both the subjective and objective somatic restlessness. Patients with akathisia may usually experience an inner tension, discomfort, irritation, anxiety, or irresistible urge to move various parts of their bodies. Akathisia appears objectively as psychomotor agitation, such as continuous pacing, rocking from foot to foot, or the inability to sit still. Akathisia is typically witnessed in a few hours to days after medication administration. This side effect can be seen in up to 20 to 25% of patients treated with conventional agents. Akathisia is frequently cited as a reason for poor drug compliance, since it is often extremely distressing to patients. It can also result in dysphoria and aggressive or suicidal behavior.

The treatment of acute EPS depends on the specific side effect. Dystonia can be quickly and successfully treated with an intramuscular injection of an anticholinergic (i.e., benztropine, diphenhydramine). The initial treatment of parkinsonian side effects is lowering the dose of antipsychotic. If an adequate response is not achieved, adding an anticholinergic, or amantadine (a weak dopamine agonist), may be efficacious. If symptoms persist, switching to an second-generation antipsychotic or a low-potency conventional antipsychotic should be considered. Akathisia is less responsive to treatment than are other acute EPS. The first step of the treatment of akathisia is lowering the antipsychotic dose. The next step is individual trials of beta-adrenergic blockers (i.e., propranolol), and benzodiazepines (i.e., lorazepam and clonazepam).

## Tardive Dyskinesia and Other Tardive Syndromes

TD is a repetitive, involuntary, hyperkinetic movement disorder caused by sustained exposure to antipsychotic medication. TD is characterized by choreiform movements, tics and grimaces of the oro-facial muscles, and dyskinesia of distal limbs, often the paraspinal muscles, and occasionally the diaphragm. Younger patients with TD tend to exhibit slower athetoid movements of the trunk, extremities, and neck. In addition to the more frequently observed oro-facial and choreoathetoid signs of TD, tardive dystonias (sustained abnormal postures or positions) and tardive akathisia (persistent subjective and/or objective signs of restlessness) have been described. The abnormal movements of TD are usually increased with emotional arousal and are absent when the individual is asleep. According to the diagnostic criteria proposed by Schooler and Kane, the movements should be present for at least four weeks, and exposure to antipsychotic drugs should have totaled at least three months. The onset of the abnormal movements should occur either while the patient is receiving an antipsychotic agent or within a few weeks of discontinuing the offending agent.

Prevalence surveys indicate that mild forms of TD occur in approximately 20% of patients who receive chronic treatment with conventional antipsychotic medication. A major prospective research demonstrates that the cumulative incidence of TD is 5% in the first year, 10% the second year, 15% the third year, and 19% the fourth year in a patient who receives a typical neuroleptic. Prevalence rates of TD may exceed 50% in high-risk groups, such as the elderly. The reported prevalence of tardive dystonia is around 1.5 to 4%. Among the most significant predictors of TD are older age, female gender, presence of EPS, diabetes mellitus, affective disorders, and certain parameters of neuroleptic exposure such as dose and duration of therapy.

All first-generation antipsychotic agents are associated with a risk of TD. Studies of newer antipsychotics suggest that TD liability is much lower with the second-generation agents, and clozapine is associated with a substantially lower risk for development of TD than other antipsychotic medications. A double-blind, random assignment study of 1,714 patients found a 0.52% long-term risk of TD with olanzapine treatment, as compared to a 7.45% risk with haloperidol. Another published double-blind randomized study showed a significantly lower risk of TD in olanzapine-treated patients (1%) than haloperidol-treated schizophrenic patients (4.6%). In a double-blind, randomized 1-year study comparing risperidone to haloperidol, the rate of TD was 0.6% in the risperidone group and 2.7% in the haloperidol group. Among a sample of geriatric patients, a lower incidence of TD in patients treated with risperidone than in those treated with haloperidol, at least over a 9-month period, has been reported. The rate of TD with risperidone has been reported to be low (0.6%) for doses currently used (2–8 mg/day). The incidence of TD with quetiapine is preliminarily reportedly low or virtually non-existent, although this remains to be demonstrated prospectively. The risk of TD with ziprasidone and aripiprazole is not known but is expected to be similarly low.

For most patients, TD does not appear to be progressive or irreversible. The onset of TD often tends to be insidious with a fluctuating course. With time, TD will either stabilize or improve even if the antipsychotic medication is continued, although there are reports of TD worsening during continued drug therapy. After discontinuation of antipsychotic medication, a significant proportion of patients with TD will have remission of symptoms, especially if the TD is of recent onset or the patient is young. Unfortunately, withdrawal of antipsychotic agents is seldom an option for patients with serious psychosis.

The American Psychiatric Association Task Force on TD has issued a report in which a number of recommendations were made for preventing and managing TD. These include (1) establishing objective evidence that antipsychotic medications are effective for an individual; (2) using the lowest effective dose of antipsychotic drugs; (3) prescribing cautiously for children, elderly patients, and patients with mood disorders; (4) examining patients on a regular basis for evidence of TD; (5) considering alternatives to antipsychotic drugs, obtaining informed consent, and also considering a reduction in dosage when TD is diagnosed; and (6) considering a number of options if the TD worsens, including discontinuing the antipsychotic medication, switching to a different drug, or considering a trial of clozapine.

Although a large number of agents have been studied for their therapeutic effects on TD, there is no definitive drug treatment for it. Second-generation antipsychotics, in particular clozapine, have been used in clinical practice to treat TD, but there have been no adequately controlled trials to date to support this practice. It has been suggested that second-generation antipsychotics should be used as first-line treatment for patients who have TD or are at risk for TD. Guidelines for treating TD recommend using second-generation agents for mild TD symptoms, and clozapine or a newer agent for more severe symptoms.

## Neuroleptic Malignant Syndrome

Neuroleptic malignant syndrome (NMS) is characterized by the triad of rigidity, hyperthermia, and autonomic instability in association with the use of an antipsychotic medication. NMS is often associated with elevation of creatine kinase (greater than 300 U/mL), leukocytosis (greater than $15,000 \, mm^3$), and change in level of consciousness. NMS can be of sudden and unpredictable onset, usually occurring early in the course of antipsychotic treatment, and can be fatal in 5 to 20% of untreated cases.

The incidence of NMS varies from 0.02 to 3.23%, reflecting differences in criteria. Prevalence rates are unknown, but are estimated to vary from 1 to 2% of patients treated with antipsychotic medication. The relative risk of second-generation antipsychotics for NMS is likely to be lower, but conclusive data are not yet available. NMS has been reported with clozapine, risperidone, olanzapine, and quetiapine. Proposed risk factors include prior episode of NMS, younger age, male gender, physical illness, dehydration, use of high-potency antipsychotics, rapid dose titration, use of parenteral (IM) preparations, and pre-existing neurological disability.

If NMS is suspected, the offending antipsychotic agent should be discontinued and supportive and symptomatic treatment started. Both dantrolene and dopamine agonists such as bromocriptine have also been used in the treatment of NMS. These agents, however, have not shown greater efficacy compared to supportive treatment.

The usual course of treatment is between 5 and 10 days. Long acting depot preparations will prolong recovery time. After several weeks of recovery, treatment may be cautiously resumed with a different antipsychotic medication with gradually increased doses.

## Endocrine and Sexual Effects

All standard antipsychotic drugs elevate serum prolactin levels by blocking the tonic inhibitory actions of dopamine on lactotrophic cells in the pituitary. Among second-generation antipsychotics, risperidone and amisulpride can produce dose-dependent hyperprolactinemia to a greater extent than first-generation antipsychotics, whereas clozapine, olanzapine, ziprasidone, and quetiapine do not cause a sustained elevation of prolactin above normal levels. Aripiprazole, being a partial DA agonist, produces no elevation of prolactin and even suppresses prolactin levels slightly. Hyperprolactinemia in women can lead to menstrual disturbances, including anovulatory cycles and infertility, menses with abnormal luteal phases, or frank amenorrhea and hypoestrogenemia. Women have also reported decreased libido and anorgasmia, and there are reports of increased long-term risk of osteoporosis although this is controversial. Antipsychotic-induced gynecomastia has been reported in 3% of women and 6% of men. Galactorrhea occurs in 2.7% of men and 10 to 50% of women. The major effects of hyperprolactinemia in men are loss of libido, impotence, hypospermatogenesis, and erectile or ejaculatory disturbances. Although amisulpride and risperidone cause significant elevations of prolactin levels, a number of studies have found only a small incidence of sexual dysfunctions in patients treated with these drugs. This may be due to the fact that these reports have relied on spontaneous reporting of sexual side effects. In a drug monitoring study, in which side effects profiles of haloperidol and clozapine were investigated, a significantly higher frequency of sexual disturbances have been found. Using a side effect rating scale, it was shown that the prevalence of these adverse events was high during the first weeks of the study. However, side effects usually remitted spontaneously despite continuous treatment in the majority of patients.

## Metabolic Effects

Various degrees of weight gain have been recognized as a common problem with conventional antipsychotic medications. Weight gain is an important issue in the management of patients, because this adverse effect may be associated with non-compliance and certain medical illnesses, such as diabetes mellitus, cardiovascular disease, certain cancers, and osteoarthritis.

Differences have been discovered among second-generation antipsychotics with respect to their ability to induce weight gain (Table 1-4). A recent meta-analysis, which estimates the weight change after 10 weeks of treatment at a standard dose, demonstrated that mean increases were 4.45 kg for clozapine, 4.15 kg for olanzapine, 2.10 kg for risperidone, and 0.04 kg for ziprasidone. The long-term risk of weight gain with quetiapine appears to be less than that with olanzapine and clozapine. Short-term weight gain (2.16 kg over 10 weeks) with quetiapine appears comparable to risperidone. Ziprasidone has been associated with minimal weight gain, which could distinguish it among other second-generation antipsychotics. Similarly, aripiprazole appears to cause little or no weight gain. During long-term treatment, clozapine and olanzapine have the largest effects on weight gain; risperidone produces intermediate weight gain; quetiapine and ziprasidone produce the least weight gain. Weight gain does not appear to be dose-dependent, tends to plateau between 6 and 12 months after initiation of treatment, and is mainly due to an increase in body fat. The mechanism by which weight gain occurs during treatment with antipsychotics is poorly understood, but the broader receptor affinities of the agents and their antagonism of histamine $H_1$ and serotonin 5-$HT_{2C}$ receptors have been implicated. There is currently no standard approach to the management of weight gain induced by antipsychotic medication. Patient education prior to initiating treatment should be provided, and regular exercise should be encouraged in all patients receiving antipsychotic medication. Switching to other second-generation antipsychotics with fewer propensities for producing weight gain may be the most efficient way to deal with antipsychotic-induced weight gain.

Abnormalities in peripheral glucose regulation and diabetes mellitus (DM) occur more commonly in schizophrenic patients compared with the general population. There is growing concern with metabolic disturbances associated with antipsychotic use, including hyperglycemia, hyperlipidemia, exacerbation of existing type 1 and 2 DM, new-onset type 2 DM, and diabetic ketoacidosis. A number of case reports have implicated both clozapine and olanzapine in the emergence of non-insulin-dependent (type 2) DM and diabetic ketoacidosis. There are fewer reports describing an association between DM and quetiapine or risperidone, but these drugs do appear to have this side effect potential albeit to a lesser degree. In contrast there are many fewer reports for ziprasidone and arip-iprazole which suggests they may have less or no metabolic side effect liability. The limited reporting for ziprasidone may be related to the relatively limited use of the agent at the present time. Although no clear mechanism of action of the second-generation agents has been established, significant weight gain or antagonism of specific serotonin receptor subtypes may contribute to the development of these abnormali-ties. Physicians employing second-generation agents should routinely monitor weight, fasting blood glucose, and lipid profiles.

## Cardiovascular Effects

Orthostatic hypotension is usually seen with low-potency conventional antipsychotic agents (e.g., chlorpromazine or thioridazine) and clozapine through alpha-l-adrenergic antag-onism. Among the first-line second-generation antipsychotics, quetiapine has the greatest potential for inducing orthostasis although all agents have this potential. Orthostasis is most likely to occur during the first few days after initiation of treatment, or when increasing the dose of medications; most patients develop tolerance to it in the following four to six weeks. Elderly patients are particularly vulnerable to this side effect and it may predispose them to falls and increase the incidence of serious injuries or fractures. A gradual upward titration of dosage may help to reduce the risk of hypotension, and patients should be advised to change posture slowly.

Tachycardia may occur as a result of the anticholinergic effects of antipsychotic medications on vagal inhibition, or secondary to orthostatic hypotension. Clozapine produces the most pronounced tachycardia; approximately 25% of patients will have a sinus tachycardia with an increase of about 10 to 15 beats per minute. Although quetiapine has virtually no cholinergic activity, tachycardia is a possible side effect, perhaps secondary to its adrenergic effects on blood pressure. Most patients will develop tolerance to this side effect over time. If tachycardia is sustained or becomes symptomatic, an electrocardiogram (ECG) should be obtained. Low doses of a peripherally acting beta-blocker such as atenolol can be useful to treat medication-induced tachycardia without hypotension.

ECG changes are observed with many antipsychotic agents. Chlorpromazine may cause prolongation of the QT and PR intervals, ST depression, and T-wave flattening or inversion, and thioridazine may cause QT and T-wave changes. These effects rarely cause clinically relevant symptoms within therapeutic dose ranges.

Ziprasidone has very specific recommendations in the package insert as to the types of patients it should not be used in. Needless to say, antipsychotics that lead to QTc-prolongation must not be combined with other drugs that have similar effects. The effect of many but not all antipsychotic drugs on the QT interval appears to be dose-related. Several antipsychotic drugs have infrequently been associated with malignant arrhythmias such as *torsade de pointes*. To date, *torsade de pointes* has not been reported following therapeutic doses or overdose with ziprasidone or other second-generation antipsychotics.

Sudden unexplained deaths have been rarely reported with therapeutic doses of antipsychotic drugs, and such deaths could result from cardiac arrhythmias in the absence of another explanation. There is, however, currently no evidence that antipsychotic drugs are associated with an increased prevalence of sudden deaths due to cardiac events, although a number of case reports and case series concerning death following cardiomyopathy, potentially induced by clozapine are a matter of concern.

## Gastrointestinal Effects

The anticholinergic effects of antipsychotic medications can induce dry mouth and constipation as well as tachycardia, urinary retention, and blurring of vision. These adverse effects are relatively commonly encountered with low-potency first-generation antipsychotics and may be dose related. In cases of more serious gastrointestinal adverse events, such as paralytic ileus, which has been reported following treatment with clozapine, medication must be discontinued immediately and relevant medical or surgical interventions may become necessary. Anticholinergic manifestations are common with poisoning from clozapine and olanzapine.

## Hepatic Effects

Asymptomatic mild, transient, and reversible elevations of liver enzyme levels occur infrequently with both first- and second-generation antipsychotic drugs. These abnormalities usually occur during the first three months of treatment, are idiosyncratic, and seldom a serious concern. Rarely, symptomatic hepatotoxicity (cholestatic or hepatitic) may be associated with second-generation antipsychotics; in these cases, the offending medication should be discontinued. Recovery occurs in up to 75% of patients within two months; 90% recover within one year. Patients taking antipsychotics who have nausea, fever, abdominal pain, and rash should have their liver function evaluated to exclude hepatotoxicity. Since antipsychotic-induced jaundice is infrequent, other etiologies should be ruled out before the cause is judged to be antipsychotic treatment.

## Hematological Effects

Antipsychotic medications may cause blood dyscrasias, including neutropenia, leukopenia, leukocytosis, thrombopenia, and agranulocytosis. Leukopenia, usually transient, commonly occurs early in treatment, and resolves spontaneously. Chlorpromazine has been associated with benign leukopenia, which occurs in up to 10% of patients. This phenomenon is even more common following clozapine administration.

Agranulocytosis (granulocyte count less than $500/mm^3$) is a fatal side effect of antipsychotic drugs. The risk of agranulocytosis with clozapine is 1% and is greatest early in treatment, usually within the first 8 to 12 weeks of treatment. It tends to occur slightly more often in women, the elderly, and young patients (less than 21 years old). Agranulocytosis from clozapine is usually reversible if the drug is withdrawn immediately. Olanzapine is not associated with severe agranulocytosis. Despite these encouraging studies, there are a number of case studies reporting agranulocytosis during treatment with olanzapine (and quetiapine) in patients who had suffered this adverse event during previous clozapine exposure.

Before initiating treatment with clozapine, patients in the USA must be registered in a program that ensures that they receive weekly monitoring of their white blood cell (WBC) count during the first six months of treatment. Current guidelines require weekly monitoring for one month after the termination of clozapine treatment. Guidelines on the use of clozapine vary between different countries.

## Other Side Effects

Sedation is the single most common side effect among low-potency conventional antipsychotics, as well as clozapine, zotepine, and quetiapine. Although sedation is often beneficial at the beginning of treatment to calm down an anxious or aggressive patient, it usually impairs functioning during long-term treatment. Most patients usually develop tolerance over time, or it may be possible to minimize sedation by dose reduction or by shifting most of the medication to night to reduce daytime sleepiness.

Antipsychotic medications can lower the seizure threshold to some degree. Seizure is more common with low-potency first-generation antipsychotics and clozapine. Clozapine is associated with dose-related increase in seizures. For example, doses of clozapine below 300 mg/day have been found to have a seizure rate of about 1%, doses between 300 and 600 mg/day have a seizure rate of 2.7%, and doses above 600 mg/day have a rate of 4.4%. Strategies to reduce the risk for seizures include slower dose titration, a lower dose, and the addition of an anticonvulsant agent (i.e., valproic acid).

## DRUG INTERACTIONS AND ANTIPSYCHOTIC AGENTS

Most antipsychotics are metabolized by hepatic microsomal oxidases (cytochrome P450 system); the major isoenzyme systems involved are CYP1A2, CYP2C19, CYP2D6, and CYP3A4. Induction or inhibition of these enzymes by other drugs may occasionally produce clinically important drug interactions. Table 1-5 summarizes clinically significant pharmacokinetic drug interactions involving second-generation antipsychotic drugs. SSRI's, particularly fluoxetine and paroxetine, can increase plasma concentrations of antipsychotic medications by inhibiting CYP2D6 and decreasing the clearance of antipsychotics, possibly leading to toxicity. Conventional antipsychotic drug clearance can be decreased by 50% with concurrent administration of certain heterocyclic antidepressants, beta-blockers, some antibiotic/antifungal agents, and cimetidine. Clozapine toxicity has occurred following co-administration with the CYP1A2 inhibitors cimetidine, erythromycin, and fluvoxamine.

Quetiapine, ziprasidone, and aripiprazole toxicity can be caused by inhibitors of CYP3A4 such as erythromycin, fluoxetine, nefazadone, and protease inhibitors.

In contrast, drugs such as carbamazepine, phenobarbital, and phenytoin can reduce plasma concentrations of antipsychotic drugs by increasing the metabolism of the antipsychotic agent. For example, carbamazepine, commonly combined with antipsychotic medications, can reduce the plasma concentration of haloperidol by 50%. Anticonvulsants, however, may not have a significant effect on the metabolic clearance of olanzapine or risperidone as they are not substantially metabolized through CYP3A4. Cigarette smoking increases drug clearance for many antipsychotic drugs, including clozapine and olanzapine. The clearance rate of clozapine and olanzapine are increased by 20 to 50%.

■ **TABLE 1-5.** Pharmacokinetic Drug Interactions Involving Second-Generation Antipsychotic Agents

| DRUG AND CYTOCHROME P-450 ISOENZYME(S) | INHIBITORS | INDUCERS |
|---|---|---|
| **Clozapine** | | |
| 1A2 | Fluoroquinolones, fluvoxamine | Smoking, PAHs[a] |
| 3A4 | Erythromycin, ketoconazole, ritonavir, sertraline,[b] cimetidine | Rifampin, carbamazepine, phenytoin, barbiturates |
| 2D6 | Ritonavir, quinidine, risperidone,[b] fluoxetine,[b] sertraline[b] | None |
| **Risperidone** | | |
| 2D6 | Paroxetine, fluoxetine | Rifampin, carbamazepine, phenytoin, barbiturates |
| **Olanzapine** | | |
| 1A2 | Fluvoxamine | Smoking, PAHs, carbamazepine |
| 2D6 | None | Phenytoin |
| **Quetiapine** | | |
| 3A4 | Ketoconazole, erythromycin | Rifampin, carbamazepine, phenytoin, barbiturates |
| **Ziprasidone** | | |
| 3A4 | Ketoconazole, erythromycin | Rifampin, carbamazepine, phenytoin, barbiturates |
| | None | None |
| **Aripiprazole** | | |
| 3A4 | Ketoconazole, erythromycin | Rifampin, carbamazepine, phenytoin, barbiturates |
| 2D6 | Paroxetine, fluoxetine | None |

[a]PAHs, polycyclic aromatic hydrocarbons.
[b]Case reports of mild to moderate elevations in serum concentration.

Adapted from Worrel JA, Marken PA, Beckman SE, et al. (2000) Atypical antipsychotic agents: A critical review. *Am J Health Syst Pharm* 57, 238–255.

Other common interactions are:

- Antacids: can decrease the absorption of the antipsychotic agent from the gut.
- Antipsychotics: can antagonize the effects of dopamine agonists or levodopa when these drugs are used to treat parkinsonism
- Antipsychotic agents: may also enhance the effects of CNS depressants such as analgesics, anxiolytics, and hypnotics.
- Doses of pre-anesthetic medication or general anesthetics may need to be reduced.

## Antipsychotic Medications and Pregnancy

Most antipsychotic agents readily cross the placenta and are secreted in breast milk to some degree. There is little data to demonstrate whether prenatal exposure to antipsychotic agents is linked to spontaneous abortion, congenital malformations, carcinogenesis, intrauterine growth retardation, or behavioral teratogenicity.

Fetal exposure over the course of pregnancy may affect development of the dopamine system; the benefits of controlling psychotic symptoms during pregnancy versus the possible risks to the mother and the fetus of withdrawing treatment and the risks to the fetus of continuing treatment must be considered.

There is no evidence that second-generation antipsychotics are teratogenic in humans. However, if possible, use of antipsychotic medication should be avoided during the first trimester, especially between weeks six and ten, unless the patient's psychosis places the mother and/or her fetus at significant risk. Antipsychotic medications may be relatively safe during the second and third trimesters of pregnancy.

If a first-generation antipsychotic is used, high-potency agents appear to be preferable for first-line management, due to a lower propensity to cause orthostasis. Low doses should be given, administration of antipsychotic medication should be as brief as possible, and the medication should be discontinued five to ten days before delivery to minimize the chances of the newborn experiencing EPS. This notion, however, has been re-evaluated, since discontinuation of medication before delivery may put the mother at risk for decompensation. Anticholinergic agents should also be avoided during pregnancy, especially for the first trimester. Since antipsychotics are also secreted into breast milk, the infants should not be breast-fed if the mother resumes antipsychotic medication postpartum.

## ADDITIONAL READING

1. Lieberman JA, Stroup TS, McEvoy JP, Swartz MS, Rosenheck RA, Perkins DO, Keefe RS, Davis SM, Davis CE, Lebowitz BD, Severe J, Hsiao JK: Effectiveness of antipsychotic drugs in patients with chronic schizophrenia. *New England Journal of Medicine* 2005; 353(12):1209–1223

2. Miyamoto S, Duncan GE, Marx CE, Lieberman JA: Treatments for schizophrenia: a critical review of pharmacology and mechanisms of action of antipsychotic drugs. *Molecular Psychiatry* 2005; 10(1):79–104

3. Lehman AF, Lieberman JA, Dixon LB, McGlashan TH, Miller AL, Perkins DO, Kreyenbuhl J; American Psychiatric Association; Steering Committee on Practice Guidelines: Practice guideline for the treatment of patients with schizophrenia, second edition. *American Journal of Psychiatry* 2004; 161(2 Suppl):1–56

4. Miyamoto S, Aoba A, Duncan GE, Lieberman JA: Acute Pharmacological Treatment of Schizophrenia. In: *Schizophrenia*, Second Edition. Blackwell Publishing, Oxford, 2002

5. Miyamoto S, Duncan GE, Goff DC, Lieberman JA: Therapeutics of Schizophrenia. In: *Neuropsychopharmacology The Fifth Generation of Progress.* Lippincott Williams & Wilkins, Philadelphia, pp. 775–807, 2002

6. Schooler NR, Kane JM: Research diagnosis for tardive dyskinesia. *Arch. Gen. Psychiat.* 1982; 39:486–487.

# 2

# ANTIDEPRESSANTS

## INTRODUCTION

The use of antidepressants in the treatment of depression
remains the best-understood use of these medications; however,
there is a growing list of other indications for antidepressants,
including panic disorder (PD), obsessive–compulsive disorder
(OCD), bulimia and posttraumatic stress disorder (PTSD).
Many of these illnesses respond best to combination treatment modalities that include medication and various forms of
psychotherapy.

## PHARMACOLOGY

The first antidepressant was the monoamine oxidase inhibitor
(MAOI), iproniazid, initially licensed as an antituberculosis
drug. This was soon followed by the tricyclic antidepressant
(TCA), imipramine. Although both were developed in the
early 1950s, they represented different paths of discovery:
iproniazid was the result of clinical and laboratory collabora-
tion, whereas imipramine's introduction was largely based on
clinical observation.

Within the past 25 years, similarly efficacious tricyclic and
heterocyclic antidepressants have been developed but with
varying side-effect profiles. A new direction in antidepressant
pharmacology began in 1987 with the discovery and

*Handbook of Psychiatric Drugs*   Jeffrey A. Lieberman and Allan Tasman
© 2006 John Wiley & Sons, Ltd

marketing of fluoxetine, the first antidepressant selective for serotonin reuptake blockade. Beyond selective serotonin reuptake inhibitors (SSRIs), the latest offerings in antidepressant pharmacology include agents that act at multiple neurotransmitter levels.

In evaluations of the many antidepressants available, the focus has generally been on the agent's side-effect profile and ease of administration. Despite many efforts in this area, there is no conclusive evidence to demonstrate the clinical superiority of any one group of agents.

## Mechanisms of Action

All known antidepressants affect monoamine neurotransmission.

MAOIs inhibit the activity of monoamine oxidase, resulting in a decrease in the breakdown of dopamine, serotonin, and norepinephrine in the synapse, thus increasing the amount of these neurotransmitters available for release and synaptic transmission. MAOIs are highly effective antidepressants and anxiolytics but are rarely used due to dietary restrictions that must be adhered to in order to avoid tyramine-induced hypertensive crises.

TCAs block presynaptic reuptake of norepinephrine and serotonin to various degrees. Several are related by metabolism, thus the tertiary amines amitriptyline and imipramine are metabolized to the secondary amines nortriptyline and desipramine respectively. All act through reuptake inhibition and are generally selective for the norepinephrine transporter; several, however, have equal or greater affinity for the serotonin transporter. The TCAs were the drugs of choice for depression through the 1980s. Though effective, their nonselective actions on cholinergic, histaminergic, and presynaptic adrenergic receptors resulted in a number of side effects.

SSRIs were first introduced in the late 1980s, and rapidly eclipsed the TCAs as the drugs of choice for depression. There are subtle differences between compounds, mainly in terms of their half-life, their potency for reuptake inhibition, and their affinity for some other receptors. As SSRIs more selectively affect reuptake, with few effects on the adrenergic, histaminergic, and cholinergic systems, side effects have been reduced.

The selective norepinephrine reuptake inhibitors (NRIs) such as reboxetine (not available in the US) or atomoxetine share a similar mechanism with the SSRIs, but act on the norepinephrine transporter and have little affinity for the serotonin transporter.

Several other second-generation agents, sometimes referred to as "atypical antidepressants", were introduced during the same period as the SSRIs. These include bupropion, which seems to exert primarily a dopaminergic effect, and trazodone, which is structurally related to the TCAs but has a primary serotonergic mechanism.

Of the serotonin receptors, 5-hydroxytryptamine type 1A ($5\text{-HT}_{1A}$) appears most related to the therapeutic effects of antidepressants, and this receptor influences norepinephrine, dopamine, acetylcholine, neuropeptides, other serotonin receptors, and probably beta-receptor downregulation.

The so-called third-generation antidepressants include serotonin–norepinephrine reuptake inhibitors (SNRIs – venlafaxine, milnacipran and duloxetine), mixed serotonin antagonist/reuptake inhibitors (nefazodone and trazodone) and the mixed serotonin/noradrenaline antagonist mirtazapine. SNRIs have equal affinity for the norepinephrine and serotonin transporter. Though, like several of the TCAs, venlafaxine has multiple receptor effects, it is relatively free of the anticholinergic and antihistaminic side effects that are common with the TCAs.

Mixed serotonin antagonist/reuptake inhibitors such as nefazodone have multiple mechanisms of action, with both serotonin (as well as norepinephrine) transporter inhibition as well as antagonism of $5\text{-HT}_{2A}$ and alpha-$1$-receptors. Trazodone is similar; however, its effects are somewhat less specific.

The mixed serotonin/noradrenaline antagonist mirtazapine is unique in that it appears to work primarily through specific receptor blockade of the alpha-$2$-autoreceptors on presynaptic noradrenergic neurons, enhancing noradrenergic output. This class may exert a similar effect toward autoreceptors on serotonin neurons. Antagonism of $5\text{-HT}_2$ and $5\text{-HT}_3$ receptors may also concentrate the effect of serotonin on $5\text{-HT}_{1A}$

receptors. The antidepressants available in the US, their class, and relative costs are listed in Table 2-1.

## Pharmacokinetics

The pharmacokinetics of TCAs are complex, as reflected in the diversity of half-lives (10 to 40 hours). TCAs are primarily absorbed in the small intestine, reaching peak plasma levels two to six hours after oral administration. Absorption can be affected by changes in gut motility. The drugs are extensively metabolized in the liver on first pass through the portal system. They are lipophilic, have a large volume of distribution, and are highly protein-bound (85–95%). TCAs are metabolized to active metabolites in the liver by hepatic microsomal enzymes and excreted by the kidneys. The rate of metabolism can vary genetically; 7 to 9% of the white population are slow hydroxylators. There is a large range of elimination half-lives.

TCAs as a class have a relatively narrow therapeutic index; there is a significant risk of toxicity with blood levels of only two to six times the therapeutic level. A 1-week supply can be fatal in overdose, as blood concentrations of greater than 1000 ng/dl are correlated with prolongation of the QRS complex and arrhythmias. TCAs are commonly ingested agents by which patients successfully commit suicide by overdose.

MAOIs are also well absorbed from the gastrointestinal tract. Their short half-life of one to two hours is not particularly relevant as they bind irreversibly with MAO. Thus, the activity of these drugs depends less on pharmacokinetics and more on the synthesis of new MAO to restore normal enzyme activity. This synthesis requires approximately two weeks. This class of drugs is little used due to their potentially dangerous interactions with sympathomimetics and foods containing tyramine.

Each of the six SSRI agents (fluoxetine, paroxetine, sertraline, fluvoxamine, citalopram and its S-enantiomer escitalopram) selectively block the reuptake of serotonin presynaptically, though each drug differs structurally from the others. As a result, these agents differ in their pharmacokinetic profiles. Many SSRIs are, like the TCAs, highly protein bound though the proportions of citalopram and escitalopram that are protein-bound are 80 and 56% respectively. In contrast,

■ TABLE 2-1. Antidepressants available in the United States

| CLASS | NAME | GENERIC | HOW SUPPLIED | RECOMMENDED DOSE PER DAY* | PRICE INDEX: (DOLLAR COST OF AVERAGE DOSE/d)** |
|---|---|---|---|---|---|
| TCAs | Amitriptyline | Y | Tablets (mg): 10, 25, 50, 75, 100, 150<br>Oral solution: 10 mg/5mL IM: 10 mg/mL | 150 mg | 0.26 |
| | Imipramine | Y | Tablets (mg): 10, 25, 50 | 150 mg | 3.65 |
| | Nortriptyline | Y | Capsules (mg): 75, 100, 125, 150<br>Oral solution: 10 mg/5 mL | 75 mg | 2.66 |
| | Desipramine | Y | Capsules (mg): 10, 25, 50, 75<br>Tablets (mg): 10, 25, 50, 75, 100, 150 | 150 mg | 2.18 |
| | Amoxapine | Y | Tablets (mg): 25, 50, 100, 150 | 300 mg | 5.00 |
| | Doxepin | Y | Oral solution: 10 mg/mL<br>Capsules (mg): 10, 25, 50, 75, 100, 150 | 150 mg | 1.66 |
| | Protriptyline | N | Tablets (mg): 5, 10 | 45 mg | 7.99 |
| | Trimipramine | N | Tablets (mg): 25, 50, 100 | 150 mg | 5.00 |
| | Clomipramine | Y | Tablets (mg): 25, 50, 75 | 150 mg | 3.03 |
| | Maprotiline | Y | Tablets (mg): 25, 50, 75 | 150 mg | 1.86 |
| MAOIs | Isocarboxazid | N | Tablets: 10 mg | 30 mg | 2.45 |
| | Phenelzine | N | Tablets: 15 mg | 60 mg | 2.64 |
| | Tranylcypromine | N | Tablets: 10 mg | 40 mg | 3.94 |

■ TABLE 2-1. (Continued)

| CLASS | NAME | GENERIC | HOW SUPPLIED | RECOMMENDED DOSE PER DAY* | PRICE INDEX: (DOLLAR COST OF AVERAGE DOSE/d)** |
|---|---|---|---|---|---|
| SSRIs | Fluoxetine | Y | Oral solution: 20 mg/5 mL<br>Tablets (mg): 10, 20, 40<br>Delayed release capsules: 90 mg<br>("Prozac Weekly") | 60 mg | 1.10 |
| | Sertraline | N | Oral solution: 20 mg/mL<br>Tablets (mg): 25, 50, 100 | 100 mg | 3.02 |
| | Paroxetine | Y | Oral solution: 10 mg/5 mL<br>Tablets (mg): 10, 20, 30, 40 | 40 mg | 2.97 |
| | Paroxetine controlled release | | Controlled release tablets (mg): 12.5, 25, 37.5 | 40 mg | 3.39 |
| | Fluvoxamine | Y | Tablets (mg): 25, 50, 100 | 200 mg | 5.25 |
| | Citalopram | Y | Oral solution: 10 mg/5 mL<br>Tablets (mg): 10, 20, 40 | 40 mg | 2.65 |
| | Escitalopram | N | Oral solution: 1 mg/1 mL<br>Tablets (mg): 5, 10, 20 | 20 mg | 2.65 |

| | | | | | |
|---|---|---|---|---|---|
| Atypical | Bupropion | Y | Tablets (mg): 75, 100 | 300 mg | 2.88 |
| | Bupropion sustained release | Y | Sustained release (mg): 100, 150 | 300 mg | 3.87 |
| | Bupropion extended release | N | Extended release (mg): 150, 300 | 300 mg | 4.84 |
| | Trazodone | Y | Tablets (mg): 50, 100, 150, 300 | 100 mg | 0.22 |
| SNRI | Venlafaxine | N | Tablets (mg): 25, 37.5, 50, 75, 100 | 225 mg | 4.30 |
| | | | Extended release (mg): 37.5, 75, 150 | 225 mg | 3.77 |
| | Duloxetine | N | Tablets (mg): 20, 30, 60 | 60 mg | 3.64 |
| Mixed serotonin antagonist/ reuptake inhibitors | Nefazodone | Y | Tablets (mg): 50, 100, 150, 200, 250 | 300 mg | 3.14 |
| Mixed serotonin/ noradrenaline antagonists | Mirtazapine | Y | Tablets (mg): 15, 30, 45<br>Dissolvable tablets (mg): 15, 30, 45 | 45 mg | 0.81 |

* Recommended dose derived from Lexi-comp online.
* The price index is a rough calculation, assuming an average recommended dose for the treatment of major depression, and assuming that the most efficient dosing regimen, and least expensive tablet choice, is prescribed. When available, generic prices are used. Prices were derived from 2006 Cardinal Health wholesale price guide provided by the Pharmacy Department of the New York State Institute.

however, they have varying half-lives ranging from approximately 24 hours to several days.

All SSRIs are well absorbed and not generally affected by food administration, though sertraline is an exception to this rule – its blood level may be increased by food. All have large volumes of distribution and are extensively protein-bound. They are metabolized by hepatic microsomal enzymes and are potent inhibitors of these enzymes. The only serotonin reuptake inhibitor with an active metabolite is fluoxetine, whose metabolite norfluoxetine has a half-life of 7 to 15 days. Thus, it may take several months to achieve steady state with this agent. This is considerably longer than citalopram (half-life 1.5 days) or sertraline and paroxetine (half-lives 24 hours).

There is no correlation between half-life and time to onset. Drugs with shorter half-lives have an advantage in cases where rapid elimination is desired (e.g., in the case of an allergic reaction). Drugs with a longer half-life may also have advantages: fluoxetine, for example, has been successfully given in a once-weekly dosing during the continuation phase of treatment and a once-weekly formulation of this drug is currently available. All serotonin reuptake inhibitors are eliminated in the urine as inactive metabolites. Both fluoxetine and paroxetine are capable of inhibiting their own clearance at clinically relevant doses. As such, they have nonlinear pharmacokinetics: changes in dose can produce proportionately large plasma levels.

Citalopram and its S-enantiomer escitalopram are the most recent SSRIs to be introduced in the Untied States; The Food and Drug Administration (FDA) approved citalopram in 1998 and escitalopram in 2002. Of the available SSRIs, these are the most selective for serotonin receptor blockade; escitalopram is 100 times more potent than the R-enantiomer.

As with most other antidepressants, bupropion undergoes extensive first pass metabolism in the liver. The parent compound has a half-life of 10 to 12 hours, but has three active metabolites. One, threohydrobupropion, has a half-life of 35 hours and is relatively free in plasma (it is only 50% protein-bound). There is considerable individual variability in the levels of bupropion and its metabolites. Trazodone has a relatively short half-life of three to nine hours; as a result of this and its apparent lack of active metabolites plasma levels of trazodone can be quite variable, requiring divided dosing.

Venlafaxine has a short half-life (4 hours); however, it is available in an extended release formulation that allows once-daily dosing. It appears to have a dual effect, in which at lower doses it primarily acts on the serotonin transporter, and clinically significant norepinephrine reuptake inhibition is not seen until higher doses are used (150 mg/day and above).

Nefazodone has relatively low bioavailability, and a short half-life (2–8 hours), and thus it is usually given in twice-daily doses. Mirtazapine has a half-life of 13 to 34 hours.

Duloxetine is the second selective inhibitor of nore-pinephrine and serotonin to be introduced in the United States. Compared with venlafaxine it has relatively greater effect on 5-HT reuptake *in vitro* but the clinical significance of this difference is unclear. The half-life of duloxetine is 8–17 hours (mean 12 hours).

The SSRIs are also, to varying degrees, potent inhibitors of the P450 hepatic enzyme system. The result is increased blood levels of concomitant agents that are also metabolized by this enzymatic system. Switching from an SSRI to another antide-pressant group illustrates the clinical relevance. For example, when a patient changes from fluoxetine to venlafaxine, the inhibition of the P450 2D6 isozyme will reduce venlafaxine metabolism for several weeks. The resulting increase in the venlafaxine blood level can hasten the development of side effects. The aware clinician can avoid this by starting with a lower than usual initial dose and titrating upward slowly.

## INDICATIONS FOR USE OF ANTIDEPRESSANTS

All antidepressants are indicated for the treatment of acute major depressive episodes; there is also evidence for their use in the prevention and relapse and recurrence. In addition, a number of more minor forms of depression may also respond to antidepressant medication, including dysthymic disorder, minor depression, and recurrent brief depression.

All antidepressants appear to treat more than depressive disorders. Particularly consistent have been data showing their utility for anxiety disorders; they have begun to supplant the sedative/hypnotics for these conditions. Many other psychiatric and medical disorders have all been successfully treated with these agents.

## Panic Disorder (PD)

SSRIs are considered the first-line treatment for anxiety disorders, with good evidence of efficacy in PD. Patients are begun at low doses (e.g., 5 mg of fluoxetine), and increased slowly to an effective dose to minimize potential side effects. There is also strong evidence for the use of TCAs and moderate evidences for the use of MAOIs.

## Obsessive–Compulsive Disorder (OCD)

SSRIs show strong evidence of effectiveness in the treatment of OCD and are considered the first-line treatment option in this disorder; all agents appear equally effective. The recommended starting dose is the same as that for depression, although higher doses (60–80 mg of fluoxetine) may be required for adequate response. There is evidence for slow but continued improvement in symptoms for many months after initiation of treatment; medication should therefore be trialed for up to four months if the patient shows a partial response. There is also strong evidence for the use of the TCA clomipramide in this disorder. Augmentation with lithium may be beneficial in partial responders.

## Generalized Anxiety Disorder (GAD)

Several agents have shown efficacy in this disorder. Good evidence exists for the use of SSRIs, venlafaxine, nefazodone and mirtazapine. Both TCAs and MAOIs have also shown moderate effectiveness; MAOIs also show efficacy in other anxiety disorders.

## Social Phobias and Posttraumatic Stress Disorder (PTSD)

SSRIs and venlafaxine have shown efficacy in social phobia (or social anxiety disorder); this condition may also be at least partially responsive to TCA medications. SSRIs have shown effectiveness in PTSD.

## Bulimia

SSRIs are commonly used in the treatment of bulimia nervosa. As with OCD, there appears to be a dose–response effect, with larger doses often required.

There is strong evidence for the use of TCAs, either alone or in combination with cognitive therapy, to decrease the binging and purging of bulimic patients. MAOIs have also been reported successful in the treatment of bulimia, although the many dietary restrictions have made physicians reluctant to prescribe these agents.

## Anorexia Nervosa

The American Psychiatric Association Practice Guidelines for Eating Disorders states that medications should not be used routinely for anorexia nervosa. They should be considered after weight gain and for persistent depression. A few published controlled studies show unimpressive results, and bupropion is contraindicated because of elevated seizure risk in patients with eating disorders.

## Body Dysmorphic Disorder (BDD)

SSRIs have also shown efficacy in the treatment of BDD. It may be at least partially responsive to TCA medications, particularly those selective for serotonin. Moderate evidence exists for the use of MAOIs.

## Premenstrual Dysphoria (PMDD)

PMDD is a chronic cyclical disorder in which serotoninergic function is reduced during the luteal phase. The treatment of choice is a SSRI; either sertraline or modified-release paroxetine, taken daily or only during the luteal phase. Treatment with sertraline should be initiated at a dose of 50 mg/day and if necessary increased in increments of 50 mg/day at each menstrual cycle to a maximum of 150 mg/day if taken every day or 100 mg/day if taken during the luteal phase only. The initial dose of modified-release paroxetine is 12.5 mg/day increasing to 25 mg/day after one week if necessary.

Intermittent dosing is usually as effective as continuous administration. Beneficial effects are seen within one to two days and response rates for improvements in mood and physical symptoms are about 50 to 60%. Evidence of long-term efficacy is lacking. Specialists recommend continuing treatment until the menopause as there is evidence that stopping treatment precipitates recurrence. Nevertheless, a trial period off treatment may be worthwhile after two years if supported by the patient.

## Childhood Disorders

TCAs, especially imipramine, are indicated for the treatment of enuresis. Anxiety and phobias in children (such as separation anxiety or school phobia and ADHD) are responsive to TCAs.

Uses for SSRIs in children include repetitive-type abnormalities associated with autism and mental retardation, ADHD (as an adjunct to methylphenidate), and chronic enuresis. Bupropion has been used successfully in the treatment of ADHD in both children and adults. It may, however, exacerbate tics in attention-deficit patients with concomitant Tourette's syndrome.

## Other Psychiatric Disorders

Other indications for SSRIs may include depersonalization disorder, obsessive jealousy, pathological gambling, Tourette's syndrome, hypochondriasis, and both paraphiliac and nonparaphiliac sexual disorders.

SSRIs have shown effectiveness in a number of more complex behavioral disorders such as obesity (particularly fluoxetine in higher doses), binge eating (sertraline), substance abuse, and to alleviate certain aggressive behaviors such as impulsivity and uncontrolled anger in adults, children, and the demented elderly.

Trazodone is frequently used as a sedative in the elderly; as it can cause or worsen orthostatic hypotension, blood pressure should be monitored when used in this group. In the demented elderly, trazodone is useful in treating behavioral disorders associated with dementia.

The sedative effect of trazodone makes it useful in weaning patients from benzodiazepines and other sedative drugs.

Nefazodone has shown efficacy in treating anxiety associated with major depression. Similarly, mirtazapine has shown efficacy in anxiety symptoms in general.

## Other Medical Conditions

Migraine and cluster headaches have been responsive to both TCAs and SSRIs. Diabetic neuropathy and other pain syndromes such as facial pain, fibrositis, and arthritis have been responsive to both TCAs and SSRIs and the SNRI duloxetine. TCAs such as protriptylene have shown efficacy for sleep apnea. SSRIs have been used in the treatment of restless leg syndrome.

A full list of indications is shown in Table 2-2.

---

■ **TABLE 2-2.** Various Uses of Antidepressants

---

Major Depression
  Acute depression
  Prevention of relapse
  Other depressive syndrome
    Bipolar depression
    Atypical depression
    Dysthymia
Other Uses

**Tricyclic Antidepressants**
  Strong evidence
    Panic disorder (most)
    Obsessive–compulsive disorder (clomipramine)
    Bulimia (imipramine, desipramine)
    Enuresis (imipramine)
  Moderate evidence
    Separation anxiety
    Attention-deficit/hyperactivity disorder
    Phobias
    Generalized anxiety disorder

---

■ **TABLE 2-2.** (Continued)

Anorexia nervosa
Body dysmorphic disorder
Migraine (amitriptyline)
Other headaches
Diabetic neuropathy, other pain syndromes
   (amitriptyline, doxepin)
Sleep apnea (protriptyline)
Cocaine abuse (desipramine)
Tinnitus
Evidence for but rarely used for these disorders
   Peptic ulcer disease
   Arrhythmias

**Monoamine Oxidase Inhibitors**
Strong evidence
   Panic disorder
   Bulimia
Moderate evidence
   Other anxiety disorders
   Anorexia nervosa
   Body dysmorphic disorder

**Atypical Agents**
Trazodone
   Insomnia
   Dementia with agitation
   Minor sedative/hypnotic withdrawal
Bupropion
   Attention-deficit/hyperactivity disorder

**Serotonin Reuptake Inhibitors**
Strong evidence
   Obsessive–compulsive disorder (high-dose
   fluoxetine, sertraline)
   Bulimia (fluoxetine)
   Panic disorder
Moderate evidence
   Generalized anxiety disorder
   Obesity (high-dose fluoxetine)
   Substance abuse
   Impulsivity, anger associated with personality
   disorder
   Pain syndromes, including diabetic neuropathy
Preliminary evidence
   Obsessive jealousy

Body dysmorphic disorder
Hypochondriasis
Behavioral abnormalities associated with autism and mental retardation
Anger attacks associated with depression
Depersonalization disorder
Social phobia
Attention-deficit/hyperactivity disorder (as an adjunct)
Chronic enuresis
Paraphilic sexual disorders
Nonparaphilic sexual disorders

**Selective Serotonin Noradrenaline Reuptake Inhibitors**
Duloxetine
    Moderate evidence
        Diabetic peripheral neuropathic pain
Venlafaxine
    Moderate evidence
        Generalized anxiety disorder
        Social phobia
        Panic disorder

## DRUG SELECTION AND INITIATION OF TREATMENT FOR MAJOR DEPRESSION

On average, all antidepressants are equally effective. Without a personal or family history of response to a particular agent, side effects are the most influential factors when selecting treatment.

Both longitudinal and cross-sectional factors should be considered when selecting an antidepressant for major depression:

- What were the course, duration, and severity of any previous episodes of depression?
- Is there a history of antidepressant response?
- How well was the antidepressant tolerated?
- Is there a family member with a history of antidepressant response; if so, to which medication?
- If there is a history of antidepressant failure, were the trials of an adequate dose and duration?
- Are melancholic, atypical, or psychotic features present?

- Does the patient have a history of sensitivity to anticholinergic, histaminic, α-adrenergic, serotonergic, or noradrenergic side effects?
- Does the patient have suicidal features or a history of impulsivity that may increase the risk for potential overdose?
- Does the patient have a history of a cardiac conduction delay or recent myocardial infarction (which would contraindicate the use of TCAs)?
- Does the patient have a history of symptoms suggestive of mania (or more minor variants of manic episodes)? If so, avoid TCAs and MAOIs
- Does the patient presently take or need sympathomimetics (which would contraindicate the use of MAOIs)?
- If an antidepressant trial has failed, was the patient a partial responder or a nonresponder?
- Were any augmentation strategies employed?

## Special Considerations in the Selection of an Antidepressant

The following factors should be considered when selecting an antidepressant agent.

*Gender*  Women may have slower gastrointestinal absorption than men due to less gastric acid and slower gastric emptying. A woman's volume of distribution differs as well, given her increased ratio of adipose tissue to lean body mass. Water retention associated with the menstrual cycle may also affect the volume of distribution. Oral contraceptives can alter the hepatic metabolism of TCAs.

*Ethnic and Racial Factors*  African-Americans may be more likely than those of European descent to be slow metabolizers of antidepressant due to possible genetic differences in metabolic enzyme expression; a growing number of studies suggest that African-Americans will have higher plasma levels per dose of antidepressant. This has been primarily demonstrated with TCAs; data with SSRIs are lacking. Some data suggest that Asians are slower to metabolize nortriptyline than other groups.

The greatest concern regarding race and ethnicity is suggested in a study of prescribing practices in Westchester County (New York) mental health clinics, which found that minorities were less likely than nonminorities to be offered antidepressant treatment, independent of diagnosis.

*Age* Is the patient elderly? If so, SSRIs are indicated as half-lives and steady-state concentrations of these agents are only minimally affected by age (although paroxetine may be an exception to this).

*Comorbidities* Patients with renal impairment may require dose adjustment for many antidepressants; fluoxetine and sertraline appear to be the exception. Liver disease can increase levels of TCAs – blood levels should be monitored. SSRIs are extensively metabolized in the liver and lower doses should be given in hepatic-impaired patients. Nefazodone is not indicated due to association with hepatic injury.

*Pregnant women and nursing mothers* Clinicians must consider whether the potential benefits of treatment justify the potential risk to the fetus. The risks of untreated depression are well-described, and the risks of medication treatment during pregnancy and lactation are less well-known. In general, studies have not shown increases in fetal malformations from antidepressant exposure. Reports of withdrawal syndromes among neonates have led some experts to recommend tapering and discontinuing antidepressants 10 to 14 days before the mother's due date. Antidepressants are excreted in varying degrees in breast milk, so breastfeeding in antidepressant-treated women should be done with caution.

*Predictors of poor response* In assessing the likelihood of success, the following predictors of poor response have been identified: neurovegetative symptoms such as hypersomnia, hyperphagia, psychomotor agitation, anxiety and irritability, personality features (such as neurotic, hypochondriacal, and hysterical traits), multiple prior episodes, delusions, and psychomotor agitation.

## Initiation of Treatment

Starting doses, titration schemes, and target doses for commonly-used TCAs, MAOIs, SSRIs, and other agents are shown in Table 2-3. Once medication is initiated, it should be gradually increased to therapeutic levels by titration.

TCAs are usually started at a relatively low dose; these low doses are preferred in elderly patients. In the frail elderly, further dose reductions may be needed −50% or less of the usual starting dose.

The usual treatment plan with SSRIs is to start a patient at the lowest effective dose and increase as indicated by clinical response. An increased response in usually seen with increased dose, however the dropout rate due to side effects also increases. For children, adolescents, the elderly, and patients who find medications generally difficult to tolerate, 50% reductions in the starting doses shown in Table 2-3 are acceptable. During titration, SSRIs may temporarily increase anxiety, insomnia, or both. These side effects can be alleviated by dose reduction, short-term use of benzodiazepines for anxiety, and the addition of either hypnotics or trazodone for sleep.

With both TCAs and SSRIs there is a significant delay between initiation of medication and response; there is no reason to believe that increasing the dose beyond the therapeutic range hastens response.

Bupropion (immediate and sustained release forms) and trazodone require divided doses. In the elderly, a usual starting dose of bupropion is 100 mg/day of the sustained release preparation, then increased to 100 mg b.i.d. Single daily dosing is possible using the extended release form of bupropion.

## Therapeutic Drug Monitoring

Although blood levels are available for many antidepressants, those for imipramine, desipramine, and nortriptyline have been best established. Imipramine and desipramine appear to have a curvilinear dose–response curve with an optimal range of 150 to 300 ng/mL. Nortriptyline appears to have a therapeutic window in the range of 50 to 150 ng/mL, usually reached by doses ranging from 50–100 mg/day. These blood levels are

**■ TABLE 2-3.** Starting Dose, Titration Steps, and Target Doses for Common Antidepressants

| | STARTING DOSE | TITRATION STEPS | TARGET DOSE | DISCONTINUATION/TAPERING |
|---|---|---|---|---|
| **TCAs** | | | | |
| Amitryptyline, imipramine, doxepin, amoxapine, clomipramine, desipramine | 50–75 mg/day | ↑ of 25 mg/day every 2–3 days or weekly ↑ of 75 mg/day | 100–150 mg/day by 2nd week, 150–200 mg/day by 3rd – 4th weeks (300 mg/d for amoxapine) | Taper all TCAs at a rate of 25–50 mg/day every 2–3 days |
| Nortriptyline | 25–50 mg/day | ↑ by 50 mg/week in young pts, 25 mg/week in elderly | 50–100 mg/day | |
| Protriptyline | 10–15 mg/day | ↑ by 5–10 mg/week | 60 mg/day | |
| **MAOIs** | | | | |
| Phenelzine | 30 mg/day | ↑ by 15 mg after 3 days, then weekly ↑ of 15 mg/day | 45–90 mg/day | |
| Tranylcypromide | 20 mg/day | ↑ by 10 mg after 3 days, then daily ↑ of 10 mg after 1 week | 30–60 mg/day | |
| Isocarboxazid | 20 mg/day | ↑ by 10 mg after 3 days | 30 mg/day | |

**■ TABLE 2-3.** (Continued)

| | STARTING DOSE | TITRATION STEPS | TARGET DOSE | DISCONTINUATION/TAPERING |
|---|---|---|---|---|
| **SSRIs** | | | | |
| Fluoxetine | 10–20 mg/day | ↑ in 10–20 mg increments | 60 mg/day 80 mg/d for OCD and bulimia nervosa | Abrupt discontinuation acceptable due to long half-life |
| Paroxetine | 10–20 mg/day | ↑ in 10–20 mg increments | 40 mg/day | Taper these SSRIs over 7–10 days |
| Paroxetine controlled release | 12.5–25 mg/day | ↑ in 12.5–25 mg increments | 50 mg/day | |
| Citalopram | 10–20 mg/day | ↑ in 10–20 mg increments | 40 mg/day | |
| Sertraline | 25–50 mg/day | ↑ in 25–50 mg increments | 50–150 mg/day for depression, 150–200 mg/day for OCD and bulimia nervosa | |
| Fluvoxamine | 50 mg/day at bedtime | ↑ in 50 mg increments | 100–200 mg/day | |
| Escitalopram | 10 mg/day | ↑ in 10 mg increments | 20 mg/day | |

## 'Atypical' antidepressants

| | | |
|---|---|---|
| Trazodone | 50–100 mg/day (requires divided doses) | ↑ in 50 mg increments | 150–300 mg/day (dose not to exceed 400 mg/day outpatient, 600 mg/day inpatient) |
| Bupropion sustained release | 100 mg/day for several days then b.i.d. | ↑ by 100–150 mg increments | 300 mg/day (max 450 mg/day) |
| Bupropion extended release | 150 mg/day | | |

## 3rd Generation

| | | |
|---|---|---|
| Venlafaxine extended release | 37.5 mg/day | ↑ to 75 mg/day within 4–7 days, then by 75 mg/day every 4 days | 225 mg/day (max 300–450 in some patients) |
| Duloxetine | 20 mg b.i.d. | ↑ by 20 mg increments | 20 mg or 30 mg twice daily or 60 mg once daily |
| Mirtazapine | 15 mg/day | ↑ by 15 mg increments | 15–45 mg/day (max 60 mg/day) |
| Nefazodone | 100 mg b.i.d. | ↑ by 100–200 mg/week | 300–600 mg/day |

nominal, as some patients do respond above or below these ranges, and blood level monitoring should not be a substitute for clinical observation.

Drug levels have not been well established for the MAOIs and the serotonin reuptake inhibitors. For the latter compounds there are numerous speculations about possible dose–response curves, including linear and "therapeutic window" models.

## Early, or Pre-response, Period

Patients should initially be followed weekly to judge their response to treatment and manage the side effects of the various medications; given realistic time and economic constraints, such contacts may at times be by telephone.

Side effects are a primary reason for treatment non-adherence, and patients may be more inclined at this early phase to simply discontinue medication rather than to first discuss it with their physician. It is inevitable that patients will experience some side effects from their medications. Patients are able to tolerate side effects better when they are framed in a positive light—as a sign that the drug is present in their system.

Strategies for reduction of side effects include:

- SSRIs, through scored tablets or liquid preparations, can be begun at 25–50% of normal starting dose in patients particularly sensitive to side effects. Panic disorder patients often fit into this category
- TCAs, although often given in a single-daily dose, could be divided across the day to minimize dose-related side effects
- Taking medications with food may decrease nausea
- Reminding patients that sedating medications should be taken in the evening, and activating ones in the morning
- Flexibility in time of dosing: a significant percentage of patients on SSRIs experience sedation rather than insomnia, warranting a change to evening dosing

Should intolerable side effects warrant medication change, select a medication in the same class as the first but with a different side effect profile; patients can have variable reactions to different SSRIs despite their apparent similarity. For instance, paroxetine is more sedative, and sertraline may cause more gastrointestinal distress than other SSRIs.

## Response, or Acute Treatment, Period

This period overlaps with the initial phase of treatment and continues until response is achieved, usually two to four months. The goal during this phase is to control the present symptoms of depression. It is important to differentiate between partial and complete response; complete response implies total recovery from all symptoms of depression, whereas a partial response is usually defined as a reduction in symptoms.

The time to response varies between patients. Few patients show a significant response before two weeks. The usual range for response is three to four weeks; however, it can take six weeks or longer. For patients who complete a satisfactory treatment regimen, the response rate for antidepressants is about 60 to 70%, although some of these responses will be partial. Response rates may be as high as 80% with antidepressants when an adequate dose is given for an adequate time.

## TREATMENT OF PARTIALLY RESPONSIVE AND NONRESPONSIVE PATIENTS

There is little benefit in making treatment changes before three weeks, other than to mitigate side effects. Changes in treatment strategy should be considered after the physician is satisfied that the patient has been treated with an adequate dosage of the antidepressant for an adequate time, with current medications increased to the limit of side effect tolerance.

In patients showing an inadequate response after a reasonable time, the decision is either to continue with the same medication and augment with an additional agent, or to switch medications altogether, depending on whether the patient has shown any response to the current strategy. Partial responders may be more likely to benefit from treatment augmentations, whereas patients who show no response or worsen during treatment warrant a new agent.

## Antidepressant Augmentation

Typical augmentation strategies shown in Table 2-4 include the addition of lithium carbonate, thyroid hormone, a stimulant, an atypical antipsychotic, or by the use of antidepressant combinations.

### LITHIUM AUGMENTATION
Lithium has been used successfully with most antidepressants, including TCAs, serotonin reuptake inhibitors, and bupropion, with response rates as high as 65%. The blood level of lithium necessary for adjunctive use has not been well established. It is probably best to start at a low dose (300 mg b.i.d) and increase to a therapeutic blood level (0.8 to 1.2 mEq/L) if there is no response. It may take three to six weeks for augmenting effect.

If augmentation is successful, it should be continued throughout the acute phase of treatment. This strategy can be limited by side effects and lithium's narrow therapeutic index. It is associated with hypothyroidism, tremor, increased thirst, increased urination, nausea, weight gain, and acne. Patients should be cautioned to avoid dehydration, which can precipitate toxic lithium blood levels.

### THYROID HORMONE AUGMENTATION
Starting dose is 25 μg/day of triiodothyronine, which can be increased to 50 μg/day in a week if there is no response. The trial should continue for at least three weeks. Reported response rates for thyroid augmentation are lower than those for lithium augmentation (25%). As with lithium augmentation, if there is a positive response, it occurs relatively early.

### STIMULANT AUGMENTATION
Methylphenidate and dextroamphetamine at dosages between 5 and 20 mg have been used for antidepressant augmentation, but there are few systematic data regarding the proper dose or length of treatment for this potential use.

### ANTIDEPRESSANT DRUG AUGMENTATION
Second-generation antipsychotic drugs are increasingly being used adjunctively with antidepressants for residual or treatment-resistant symptoms. APDs are generally used within their therapeutic range.

■ TABLE 2-4. Augmentation Strategies

| AGENT | DOSING STRATEGY | LENGTH OF TRIAL | REPORTED RESPONSE RATE | COMMENTS |
|---|---|---|---|---|
| Lithium carbonate | Start at 300 mg b.i.d., increase to therapeutic blood level (0.8–1.2 mEq/L) | 3–6 wks | As high as 65% | Best documented strategy; has been combined with most agents |
| Triiodothyronine | Start at 25 µg/d, may increase to 50 µg/d | At least 3 wks | At 25% | Equal to lithium in one placebo controlled trial Few systematic data |
| Stimulants (methylphenidate dextroamphetamine) | † | † | † | |
| Atypical antipsychotics | Begin with low dose (e.g., olanzapine 2.5 mg/day, aripiprazole 5 mg/day) gradually increase to full therapeutic dose if needed | † | † | Mainly open trials; controlled studies in progress |
| Combined antidepressant therapy | May need lower doses than usual (due to enzyme inhibition) † | † | † | Mainly open trials; controlled studies in progress |
| Psychotherapy | N/A | Varies by therapy | Varies by therapy | Good data for both cognitive–behavioral therapy and interpersonal therapy |

† Inadequate data.

**COMBINED ANTIDEPRESSANT THERAPY**

Open trials have supported the use of combined therapy of a TCA and a serotonin reuptake inhibitor in patients for whom either class alone has failed. When antidepressants are combined, it is important to remember that the serotonin reuptake inhibitors can potentiate TCA levels, and this should be monitored carefully. MAOIs have also been used in combination with TCAs, although this should be monitored closely given the risk of potential toxic interactions. Given the risk of a serotonin syndrome, MAOIs should not be combined with serotonin reuptake inhibitors. Bupropion is frequently added to an SSRI to enhance efficacy or to alleviate side effects such as decreased libido, fatigue, and sedation.

**NONPHARMACOLOGICAL APPROACHES**

A number of nonpharmacological augmentation options exist, particularly the concomitant use of psychotherapy. The combination of psychotherapy and medication may offer benefits that either therapy alone cannot offer, including additional efficacy as well as prevention of relapse. This has been shown to some degree for both cognitive–behavioral therapy and interpersonal therapy.

## Changing to a New Agent

Patient showing no response or whose condition deteriorates during therapy should trial an alternative single agent. Recent studies support the belief that it is best to switch to an agent of a different class, and approximately 50% of patients unresponsive to a first trial respond to an antidepressant of a different class.

When the switch involves an MAOI, sufficient time must be given for medication clearance. Although seldom used, MAOIs may be very effective in patients not responsive to other classes of antidepressants. Generally, 10 to 14 days is required for clearance of TCAs and MAOIs. Fluoxetine requires a much longer period—6 weeks—whereas sertraline and paroxetine require about two weeks when switching to an MAOI. Another alternative is changing from an SSRI medication to an SNRI. There is some evidence that SNRIs may lead to higher rates of response and remission than SSRIs.

***ECT*** ECT and other forms of stimulant therapies (e.g., vagal nerve stimulation) should be considered for patients who are non-responsive to pharmaco- and psychotherapies.

## Continuation and Maintenance Periods, and Discontinuation

### CONTINUATION PERIOD

This period usually lasts five to eight months after the end of the acute treatment period. The goal at this phase is the prevention of relapse. There is a high risk of relapse if treatment is discontinued after the acute treatment phase, with rates of 15% after six months and 22% after 12 months. The two best predictors of relapse are a high number of previous depressive episodes (greater than three predicted relapses) and underlying dysthymic disorder.

Once a patient has responded to medication, treatment should be continued for a minimum of four to six months from the point of initial response. This period should be lengthened for the patient with a history of longer depressive episodes.

In the past, it was suggested that, on achievement of euthymia, doses could be reduced. However, it is more likely that levels similar to those needed at the acute stage of treatment will be required throughout the continuation period.

### MAINTENANCE PERIOD

The goal of the maintenance period is to prevent the recurrence of depression. There are a number of reasons to consider long-term prophylactic therapy for depression rather than medication withdrawal:

1. Depression is a lifelong disease, with recurrence being the norm rather than the exception
2. As the number of acute episodes increases, the risk of future episodes increases as well, and the interval between episodes shortens
3. Each subsequent episode carries a higher morbidity and disability
4. There is a fear that treatment response may decrease with an increasing number of depressive episodes

Several factors influence the decision to maintain long-term prophylaxis for depression, including the seriousness of previous episodes, the severity of impairment caused by such episodes, the degree of response to previous treatments, and the ability of the patient to tolerate the drug. Central in the decision process is the concept of recurrent depression: that some patients are more likely than others to have a recurrence of the disease. Three previous episodes of depression make recurrent depression likely.

The best predictors of the likelihood of recurrence appear to be older age of onset and number of episodes. Long-term maintenance is the treatment of choice for the following groups of patients:

1. 50 years old or more at the time of the first depressive episode
2. 40 years old or more at first episode and have had at least one subsequent recurrence
3. Anyone who has had more than three episodes

The recommended length of maintenance therapy varies from five years of treatment to indefinite continuation. Recent studies with both acute major depression and recurrent depression have shown significantly higher relapse rates 2–3 years post-discontinuation compared with patients on maintenance treatment.

Regarding choice of agent, there are no rigorous studies comparing different antidepressants during the maintenance period. It is usually assumed that the same agent used in the acute and continuation period will also be the preferred one in the maintenance period.

Equally important in preventing recurrence of depression is the problem of maintaining adherence to medication long after the acute episode has resolved. Proper education and support will help with compliance. Toleration of side effects is important; patients are more likely to comply with agents that have more favorable side effect profiles. SSRIs or bupropion (sustained or extended release forms) are generally the best-tolerated antidepressants.

Although lower doses for prophylaxis have been recommended, there are few data to support this contention. Even though lower doses may increase compliance, full doses should be used until new information indicates otherwise.

### DISCONTINUATION OF TREATMENT

Before discontinuing treatment with an antidepressant it is important to remember that depression is often a lifelong disease with a chronic course. One should always weigh the benefits of discontinuation against the risks of recurrent depression. Patients with a single episode of acute depression and who have an onset before age 50 are the best candidates for discontinuation.

For TCAs, the usual strategy is to taper the dose at a rate of 25 to 50 mg/day every 2 to 3 days. Too rapid a decrease in dose may produce symptoms of cholinergic 'rebound' or supersensitivity (nausea, vomiting, cramps), other signs of autonomic hyperactivity (diaphoresis, anxiety, agitation, headache), and insomnia as early as 48 hours or as late as 2 weeks after discontinuation. These early symptoms may be mistaken for relapse of depression.

MAOIs may also have a withdrawal syndrome on abrupt cessation of treatment, including symptoms of psychosis; however, this is rarer than that seen with the TCAs.

Recommendations for discontinuing SSRIs depend on the particular drug. Fluoxetine has a long half-life and abrupt withdrawal should be permissible. Shorter half-life drugs, such as sertraline, citalopram, escitalopram, and paroxetine, may require a 7–10-day taper. The withdrawal syndrome with shorter-acting agents includes symptoms of fatigue, insomnia, abdominal distress, and influenza-like symptoms. The same may be true for venlafaxine and duloxetine.

A first episode of depression has a high risk of recurrence and the risk is higher in patients who have only a partial response to treatment. After discontinuation the goal is to enable early intervention if symptoms recur. The patient should be educated to recognize the symptoms of depression and seek help at an early stage.

## SIDE EFFECTS

Once the choice of an antidepressant has been made, the main goal is to maximize therapeutic effects and minimize side effects. Good preparation and reassurance of the patient is essential. Even relatively benign side effects are a major cause of treatment nonadherence; drop-out rates ranging from 7 to 44% have been reported in various studies of TCAs, and from 7 to 23% in studies of serotonin reuptake inhibitors. Common side effects for TCAs and SSRIs are shown in Table 2-5.

## Anticholinergic Effects

Common side effects include dry mouth, constipation, urinary retention, blurred vision, and less commonly narrow-angle glaucoma. These effects are usually dose-related and worse in patients with pre-existing defects.

Dry mouth can be alleviated by saliva substitutes or sugar-free hard candy, over-the-counter bulk-forming laxatives can treat the constipation caused by some agents, and the cholinergic agonist bethanechol has been used to treat anticholinergic side effects, particularly urinary hesitancy and blurred vision. The usual adult dosage is 10 to 50 mg t.i.d. or q.i.d. Pilocarpine eye drops can also be used to treat blurred vision. SSRIs in general are free from these side effects, as is buproprion, although duloxetine and paroxetine may cause mild dry mouth and constipation.

Other effects include tachycardia, impaired memory and cognition (in severe cases leading to delirium), and exacerbation of texisting tardive dyskinesia.

Rarely, in combination with other anticholinergic drugs, TCAs can precipitate a central anticholinergic delirium and confusion. Patients with psychotic depression may be at higher risk as their treatment regimen may include a TCA, a low-potency antipsychotic, and an antiparkinsonism agent. If this syndrome is suspected, a physostigmine challenge can be diagnostic and may produce a dramatic reversal. Abrupt withdrawal of TCAs can put patients at risk of cholinergic rebound. This syndrome includes gastrointestinal distress, anxiety, and autonomic instability. Whenever possible, TCA doses should first be slowly tapered and then discontinued.

## Autonomic Effects

The most frequent and treatment-limiting side effect of TCAs is orthostatic hypotension. The geriatric population is

■ **TABLE 2-5.** SSRI, SNRI and TCA Side Effects

**Side Effects of Serotonin Blockade**
Jitteriness, activation
Insomnia
Anorexia, weight loss
Nausea, vomiting, diarrhea
Sexual dysfunction
Extrapyramidal-like side effects
Increase in suicidal ideas

**Signs and Symptoms of Central Serotonergic Syndrome**
Confusion, disorientation
Headache
Autonomic instability
Lethargy
Restlessness
Abdominal cramps, diarrhea
Tremor, myoclonic jerks

**Side Effects of Norepinephrine Blockade**
Tremors
Jitteriness
Tachycardia
Diaphoresis
Augmentation of pressor effects of sympathomimetics
Sexual dysfunction

**Anticholinergic Side Effects**
Dry mouth
Constipation (rarely—paralytic ileus)
Urinary hesitancy (rarely—dystonic bladder)
Blurred vision
Sinus tachycardia
Memory impairment
Worsening of narrow-angle glaucoma

**Anticholinergic Delirium**
"Mad as a hatter": confusion, disorientation, visual hallucinations
"Hot as a hare": hyperpyrexia
"Blind as a bat": loss of visual accommodation
"Red as a beet": peripheral vasodilation
"Dry as a bone": drying of mucous membranes

From Mendelowitz AJ, Dawkins K and Lieberman JA (2000). Antidepressants. In *Psychiatric Drugs*, Lieberman JA and Tasman A (eds.) WB Saunders, pp. 44–77. © 2000, with permission from Elsevier.

especially vulnerable to falls; patients should be educated in how to change position safely. Newer TCAs such as nortriptyline and doxepin have a lower risk of this side effect. Trazodone has significant $\alpha_1$-adrenergic blockade and as a result also induces significant orthostatic hypotension.

Both SSRIs and TCAs may also cause sweating, palpitations, and increased blood pressure. Venlafaxine and duloxetine also cause sweating and tremor, and slightly increase blood pressure and heart rate; increases in blood pressure are most notable in doses of venlafaxine above 300 mg/day.

## Neurologic Effects

Several TCAs may lower the threshold for epileptic seizures, although as a class they have relatively low risk for inducing seizures. Initial doses of TCAs should be reduced in epileptic patients. Some SSRIs may increase the frequency of seizures at high dose, particularly fluoxetine at doses of 100 mg/day or more. Buproprion is the agent most likely to reduce the seizure threshold. In doses below 450 mg/d, the incidence of seizures is less than 0.5%. To avoid inducing a seizure, one should give bupropion in divided doses, with a maximum dose of 450 mg/d (400 mg/d for the extended release formulation). Seizure risk is likely to be lower with sustained or extended release forms of buproprion.

Myoclonic twitches and tremor of the tongue and upper limbs can occur in 5–10% of patients on SSRIs and less frequently with TCAs; this may respond to dose reduction or the addition of a low-dose beta blocker such as propranolol. Anxiety, nervousness, insomnia, and sedation may also occur with SSRI agents; these symptoms may respond to a dose reduction or to the short-term addition of a low-dose benzodiazepine. Insomnia is often already part of the depression; the addition of a low-dose of a sedating antidepressant such as trazodone, or a sedative–hypnotic, may allieviate symptoms in the short term. It is more common with high doses of fluoxetine. Headache may also occur with fluoxetine.

More rarely, paresthesia, ataxia, and speech blockade may occur with both TCAs and SSRIs.

There is some question as to whether SSRIs can induce extrapyramidal-like symptoms, specifically akathisia. It remains unclear whether this is actually an extrapyramidal effect or part of the agitation and anxiety that these agents can produce. The TCA amoxapine can cause extrapyramidal side effects including acute dystonic reactions, parkinsonism symptoms, akathisia, tardive dyskinesia, and neuroleptic malignant syndrome. If akathisia is suspected, dosage reduction may be required.

## Weight Gain

Both TCAs and SSRIs cause weight gain; up to 30% of patients on SSRIs experience this side effect, with increases of 8 kg or more. This is less of a concern during the acute phase of treatment, when insomnia and anorexia are often present, but they can be treatment limiting when long-term use is indicated. Medication switches to less weight-increasing medication may be helpful.

## Gastrointestinal Symptoms

Nausea, vomiting, anorexia, and diarrhea are frequent complaints with SSRIs. They are often dose and titration dependent and can be lessened by dose reduction, a slower initial titration, and having the patient take medications with food. Anorexia usually occurs only early in treatment and is not persistent. Side effects and treatment discontinuation during the early days of treatment associated with paroxetine may be reduced by prescribing the modified-release formulation Paxil CR. Compared with immediate-release tablets, this formulation significantly reduces the incidence of nausea during the first week of therapy. The most frequent adverse effect associated with both venlafaxine and duloxetine is nausea.

## Sexual Dysfunction

Every class of antidepressants is associated with some degree of sexual dysfunction. Difficulties can include problems with libido, impotence, ejaculatory dysfunction, and anorgasmy. The incidence of sexual dysfunction is as high as 30% with SSRIs. As with other side effects, some of these may be symptoms of the depression itself, and they may predate the initiation of the antidepressant trial. Treatment can include dose reduction, skipping of a dose of an SSRI with a short half-life (e.g., sertraline), or changing to an antidepressant of a different class. Anorgasmia may be treated by the addition of yohimbine or amantadine or by the use of bethanechol or cyproheptadine one to two hours before sexual activity. Decreased libido may be treated by the addition of the antidepressant bupropion; in general, this agent has the best profile with respect to sexual dysfunction. Trazodone has been associated with priapism in rare cases; this must be treated urgently to avoid long-term impairment.

## Cardiac Conduction

TCAs affect cardiac conduction; as a result, they have antiarrhythmic properties and can slow cardiac conduction. These effects are responsible for the cardiotoxicity of TCAs and their danger in overdose. TCAs do not affect cardiac output, however they should not be used in patients with a preexisting conduction delay greater than a first-degree block or in patients immediately after myocardial infarction.

## Suicide Risk

SSRIs have a very wide therapeutic index and are not lethal in overdose. This has made them especially popular in the treatment of patients with a history of impulsivity. The possibility that treatment with any type of antidepressant may increase the risk of suicide in adults is currently under active review. It is clinically prudent to limit the amount prescribed during the initiation of therapy or when patients are only partially treated. The risk of suicide attempts during these intervals is high. More than a 1-week supply of a TCA is potentially lethal in an overdose attempt.

Pooled analysis of clinical trials involving children and adolescents suggests that antidepressants are associated with suicidal thinking or behavior in about 4% of patients compared with 2% receiving placebo during the early months of treatment.

All patients treated with an antidepressant (adults as well as children and adolescents) should therefore be closely monitored during the first few months. Treatment may need to be adjusted or discontinued if depression continues to worsen or suicidal ideation emerges, especially if the symptoms are severe, abrupt in onset, or not part of the patient's presenting symptoms. Patients should be warned of this possibility and provided with information about the risk and advice on what precautions to take. They should be warned to report new or increased signs of irritability, agitation, or suicidality to a healthcare professional.

## Allergic and Hematologic Effects

TCAs are associated with exanthematous rashes in 4–5% of patients, while SSRIs have been known to cause a variety of rashes in a similar percentage of patients.

## Other Effects

TCA's can cause gynecomastia and amenorrhea in some patients, while SSRIs can cause increased prolactin levels causing mammoplasia and galactorrhea in both men and women. SSRIs have also been known to reduce blood glucose levels, though this is rare. Nefazodone has been associated with rare cases of life-threatening liver failure, and has been removed from the market in many European countries. As a result, nefazodone should not normally be considered for use before other antidepressants.

## Central Serotonergic Syndrome

Any agent that increases serotonergic function can put patients at risk of a central serotonergic syndrome. This syndrome most commonly affects patients on multiple serotonergic drugs, and involves multiple systems. The syndrome can in rare cases progress to rhabdomyolysis, acidosis, respiratory compromise, disseminated intravascular coagulation, and cardiac collapse.

## Monoamine Oxidase Inhibitors

The declining popularity of MAOIs in the United States is primarily the result of the need for dietary restrictions and the potential for serious side effects. Use of MAOIs must be limited to patients who are compliant with a tyramine-free diet and do not use any medications that contain sympathomimetic amines. A hypertensive crisis is a potentially fatal, though rare, complication of these drugs. The crisis is usually preceded by a prodrome that includes increased blood pressure, headache, stiff neck, and vomiting. Treatment needs to be immediate and may include the administration of phentolamine, 5 mg i.v.

## DRUG INTERACTIONS

The most common drug interaction with antidepressants is their influence on the metabolism of other drugs. Antidepressants are metabolized through catabolic enzymes located in a variety of places, but primarily in the smooth endoplasmic reticulum of hepatocytes: the cytochrome P450 (CYP) enzymes. Many other drugs are also metabolized through similar pathways: it is estimated that about half of all drugs prescribed depend on CYP for their metabolism.

Of these enzymes, most drugs are metabolized by the enzymes CYP3A4 (50%) and CYP2D6 (20%). Other clinically important CYP enzymes include CYP2C9, and CYP2C19 and CYP1A2, the latter which is found in the brain and may affect CNS distribution of antidepressants. A list of the enzymes and some drugs commonly affected by them is found in Table 2-6.

### Tricyclic Antidepressants

As with any combination therapy, the side effects described previously can be additive with other similar drugs. Most problematical are the anticholinergic effects of the TCAs. Such cholinergic blockade is a property shared by many other medications, including numerous over-the-counter preparations. The general sedative properties of these medications can also augment any soporific. The slowing of cardiac conduction can also potentiate other medications that produce similar effects, such as type IA antiarrhythmics and anticholinergic medications. Adrenergic receptor blockade can worsen the orthostatic hypotension caused by other medications, including vasodilators and low-potency antipsychotic medications.

■ **TABLE 2-6.** Cytochrome P-450 Isoenzymes and Common Medications Inhibiting or Inducing Them

| | INHIBITORS | INDUCERS |
|---|---|---|
| **1A2** | Cimetidine, fluoroquinolones, fluvoxamine, ticlopidine | Tobacco |
| **2C19** | Fluoxetine, fluvoxamine, ketoconazole, lansoprazole, omeprazole, ticlopidine | |
| **2C9** | Amiodarone, fluconazole, isoniazid, ticlopidine | Rifampin, secobarbital |
| **2D6** | Amiodarone, chlorpheniramine, cimetidine, clomipramine, fluoxetine, haloperidol, methadone, mibefradil, paroxetine, quinidine, ritonavir | |
| **3A4,5,7** | HIV protease inhibitors: (indinavirn, elfinavir, ritonavir, saquinavir, amiodarone, but not azithromycin) cimetidine, clarithromycin, erythromycin, fluoxetine, fluvoxamine, grapefruit juice, itraconazole, ketoconazole, mibefradil, nefazodone, troleandomycin | Carbamazepine, phenobarbital, phenytoin, rifabutin, rifampin, St. John's wort, troglitazone |

## Pharmacokinetic Effects

Absorption of TCAs can be inhibited by cholestyramine, which therefore must be given at different time intervals than the antidepressants. Specific substances reported to increase TCA levels include fluoxetine, antipsychotic medications, methylphenidate, and cimetidine. Methylphenidate has been combined with desipramine to treat attention deficits and depression in children. The combination therapy had a higher incidence of ECG changes (particularly higher ventricular rates), nausea, dry mouth, and tremor. Enzyme "inducers" that can lower tricyclic agent levels include phenobarbital and carbamazepine. The nicotine from cigarettes can also induce enzyme activity.

Guanethidine is contraindicated with TCAs, as it relies on neuronal reuptake for its antihypertensive effect. Clonidine, a presynaptic alpha-$_2$-receptor noradrenergic agonist, is also contraindicated, as it works in an antithetical fashion to tricyclic medications.

## Monoamine Oxidase Inhibitors

As with the dietary proscriptions, any medication that increases tyramine can precipitate a hypertensive crisis; such medications include numerous over-the-counter preparations for coughs, colds, and allergies. The same rule applies to sympathomimetic drugs (such as epinephrine and amphetamines or cocaine) and dopaminergic drugs such as anti-parkinsonian medications.

The combination of MAOIs and narcotics, particularly meperidine, may cause a fatal interaction. The reaction can vary from symptoms of agitation and hyperpyrexia to cardio-vascular collapse, coma, and death. A similar reaction has also been reported when propoxyphene, diphenoxylate hydrochloride, and atropine are used with MAOIs. The combination of MAOIs with agents such as SSRIs can cause the serotonin syndrome.

## Serotonin Reuptake Inhibitors

Serotonin reuptake inhibitors are potent inhibitors of the CYP2D6 pathway and can slow the metabolism of any drug that is also metabolized by that pathway. Such drugs include TCAs, carbamazepine, phenothiazines, butyrophe-nones, opiates, diazepam, alprazolam, verapamil, diltiazem, cimetidine, and bupropion. Paroxetine appears to be the most potent inhibitor of this metabolic pathway, with fluoxetine also showing high potency. Sertraline is a somewhat less potent inhibitor. These pharmacokinetic interactions are best managed with dosage adjustment. Fluoxetine, for example, can be safely used with tricyclic medications if TCA blood levels and, possibly, electrocardiograms are monitored. Although it binds more weakly to the CYP2D6, sertraline has also been reported to raise the level of TCAs significantly. In the case of bupropion, this relative increase in the blood level can increase the risk for seizures.

Particular caution should be used when a patient using multiple medications starts a serotonin reuptake inhibitor, as the interactions with other drugs can cause dangerous increases in levels. For example, in the cardiac patient, levels of warfarin should be monitored as fluoxetine has been reported to raise these levels. Several case reports exist of increased antiarrhythmic levels after introduction of fluoxetine, which resulted in potential serious bradyarrhythmias.

Fluoxetine has also been reported to raise lithium levels. The mechanism for this is not clear, as lithium is primarily excreted through the kidneys.

## Other Second-Generation Antidepressants

Few reports exist of interactions with other drugs and trazodone, although trazodone may increase levels of digoxin, phenytoin, and possibly warfarin. Bupropion causes few drug–drug interactions. The main interactions reported have occurred when bupropion is combined with another dopaminergic agent. For example, when bupropion was used with l-dopa, the combination caused excitement, restlessness, nausea, vomiting, and tremor.

## Third-Generation Antidepressants

Venlafaxine does not substantially inhibit the CYP enzyme, and is not highly protein-bound, thus it tends to have few clinically significant drug–drug interactions. Duloxetine is metabolized by 1A2 and 2D6 P450 isoenzymes, and may increase plasma levels of other antidepressants, antipsychotics, and Type 1C antiarrhythmics, such as flecainide (Tambocor). Nefazodone is highly protein-bound, and has several active metabolites. It is also a strong inhibitor of CYP3A4, and affects other drugs also metabolized by that pathway; however, it has little affinity for the CYP2D6 enzyme. Mirtazapine is highly protein-bound as well, but appears to only weakly affect the cytochrome enzymes.

## SUMMARY

There remain a number of important limitations regarding the pharmacotherapy of depression. Some of these limitations can be addressed by continued progress on current research. Other limitations await truly novel research into the mechanism of depression.

## Recommendations for the Use of Antidepressants

Allowing for the many limitations, we can generalize from available data to make the following recommendations:

1. All patients with acute major depression should be considered reasonable candidates for pharmacotherapy.
2. There is adequate evidence to make the same recommendation for other forms of depression. This is particularly true for dysthymia, and may be true for other minor forms of depression as well.
3. There is good evidence for the use of antidepressants for non-mood disorders as well, particularly the anxiety disorders.
4. There remains no strong evidence from choosing one medication over another, and treatment recommendations should be made on the basis of tolerability and, if appropriate, cost.
5. Extended treatment should be recommended both for patients with chronic depression and recurrent depression.
6. Maintenance treatment should consist of the same dose of antidepressant as used to achieve acute phase remission.
7. The exact length of maintenance treatment is not known. The decision for indefinite treatment should be a risks–benefit decision, made with the informed consent of the patient, who is entitled to be informed of the limitations in our knowledge.

### ADDITIONAL READING

1. Weissman, MM. *Treatment of Depression: Bridging the 21st Century.* American Psychiatric Press, Washington D.C., 2001
2. Potokar J, Thase M. *Advances in the Management and Treatment of Depression.* Taylor & Francis, London, 2003
3. Lieberman JA, Greenhouse J, Hamer RM, Krishnan KR, Nemeroff CB, Sheehan DV, Thase ME, Keller MB: Comparing the effects of antidepressants: consensus guidelines for evaluating quantitative reviews of antidepressant efficacy. *Neuropsychopharmacology* 2005; 30(3):445–460

4. Wong IC, Besag FM, Santosh PJ, Murray ML. Use of selective serotonin reuptake inhibitors in children and adolescents. *Drug Safety* 2004; 27:991–1000
5. Practice guidelines for the treatment of patients with major depressive disorder, Second Edition. In: American Psychiatric Association Practice Guidelines for the Treatment of Psychiatric Disorders, Compendium 2004, American Psychiatric Publishing, Arlington VA, 2004

# 3

# MOOD STABILIZERS

## INTRODUCTION

Although a wide variety of medications are employed in the treatment of bipolar disorder and related conditions, the essential ingredient in any treatment regimen is one or more mood stabilizers. By definition, these are medications which can effect at least one phase of the illness without worsening any other phases. Currently accepted mood stabilizers fall into three families: (1) lithium, (2) a subset of anti-epileptic drugs (anticonvulsants), and (3) all of the second-generation or atypical antipsychotics. Agents currently approved for the treatment of bipolar disorder are listed in Table 3-1.

Lithium was approved by the US Food and Drug Administration (FDA) in 1970, is the medication with the longest history of use for bipolar disorders, and remains a primary agent for the acute and maintenance treatment of the disorder. However, the rate of non-response to lithium is between 20 and 40%, it is less effective for bipolar depression than for mood elevation, and it possesses a relatively narrow therapeutic index. In addition, lithium is most effective in patients with classic symptom patterns (e.g., pure euphoric mania) and early in the course of illness. Patients with dysphoric and mixed episodes, rapid cyclers, patients with a history of neurologic disease, and those with comorbid substance abuse may be

*Handbook of Psychiatric Drugs*    Jeffrey A. Lieberman and Allan Tasman
© 2006 John Wiley & Sons, Ltd

■ **TABLE 3-1.** Current FDA Indications

| MEDICATION | ACUTE INDICATION | MAINTENANCE INDICATION |
|---|---|---|
| Lithium | Mania | Mania |
| Divalproex | Mania | |
| Carbamazepine | Mania* | |
| Lamotrigine | | Mania or Depression, Monotherapy |
| Olanzapine | Mania<br>Mania, Adjunct to Li and Valproate | |
| Olanzapine & Fluoxetine Comb. | Depression | |
| Quetiapine | Mania, Monotherapy<br>Mania, Adjunct to Li and Valproate | |
| Risperidone | Mania, Monotherapy<br>Mania, Adjunct to Li and Valproate | |
| Ziprasidone | Mania, Monotherapy | |
| Aripiprazole | Mania, Monotherapy | Mania, Monotherapy |

* Extended release formulation.

less likely to respond to lithium than some other mood stabilizers. Therefore, although lithium remains a mainstay of management, newer agents such as anticonvulsants and atypical antipsychotics play an increasingly important role.

Long-term prospective studies have shown that, even with conscientious medication treatment, patients with bipolar disorder are still symptomatic approximately half of the time. Despite increasing numbers of medications approved for the treatment of bipolar disorder, we still often struggle with incomplete efficacy, significant side effects, and the need to combine medications to maximize response. Residual symptoms and breakthrough episodes all too often lead to suffering, dysfunction, and loss of life. However, when the pharmacologic management of the bipolar patient is approached in an organized and systematic way, based upon updated knowledge of the strengths and limitations of specific agents, and when comorbidities are addressed and psychosocial supports bolstered, one can often see tremendous improvements.

## PHARMACOLOGY

### Chemistry

Lithium is clearly the most structurally simple psychotropic agent, with therapeutic activity residing in the lithium ion, $Li^+$. The anticonvulsants are chemically unrelated agents that are not classified by their chemistry, except for closely related agents such as carbamazepine and oxcarbazepine, or different salts such as valproate and divalproex. The chemistry of antipsychotic agents is summarized in Chapter 1.

### Mechanism of Action

The mechanism of action of anti-manic drugs is poorly understood. Whereas alterations in monoamine systems are generally believed to be critical for antidepressant response, it is not clear which neurotransmitter systems are involved in the mood stabilization. Indeed, few significant changes in neurotransmitter levels have been measured following treatment with mood stabilizers. Rather, a range of clinical and preclinical studies strongly suggests that the critical site of action for many mood stabilizers occurs at the level of intracellular second-messenger systems.

#### LITHIUM

Lithium is a monovalent cation and appears to exert its clinical effect by directly interacting with intracellular targets. At therapeutic serum concentrations, lithium is a direct competitor of magnesium at several important regulatory enzymes, including inositol-monophosphatase (IMPase), which catalyzes the rate limiting step in the phosphoinositol signaling cascade. According to the inositol depletion hypothesis, inhibition of IMPase by lithium reduces myoinositol and phosphoinositide phosphate (PIP-2), thereby reducing G protein mediated signaling, intracellular calcium mobilization and protein kinase

C (PKC) activation. Ultimately, these cascades produce wide-ranging effects on gene transcription, ion channel function and even neuronal structure and synaptic function. It has been postulated that lithium shifts the level of activation in these complex and integrated second messenger systems, providing neurons (and the circuits in which they act) with greater stability and resilience. Magnetic resonance spectroscopy studies have recently demonstrated that five days of lithium treatment significantly reduces frontal cortex myoinositol levels. In support of this system being therapeutically relevant, two PKC inhibitors, tamoxifen and riluzole, have been shown to be effective in treating bipolar mania and depression, respectively. Another enzyme directly inhibited by lithium is glycogen synthase kinase-3 (GSK-3), which has been implicated in a wide range of normal and pathological processes. GSK-3 influences transcription factors and regulators of cellular metabolism, impacting upon neuronal resilience and survival. Specific GSK-3 inhibitors are being actively studied for potential therapeutic use in Alzheimer's disease, diabetes and other disorders.

### ANTICONVULSANTS

The mechanisms by which some of the anticonvulsants stabilize mood are unknown. Valproate acts at sodium channels, at several important steps in GABA metabolism, and on the activity of histone deacetylase (which influences gene transcription). It has also be shown in preclinical studies to produce changes in the phosphoinositol pathway similar to those caused by lithium, including a reduction of PKC activity at clinically relevant serum levels.

Carbamazepine exerts a range of effects on neurotransmitter systems, increasing acetylcholine in the striatum, and decreasing dopamine and GABA turnover, and norepinephrine release. It is not clear which, if any, of these effects are relevant to its therapeutic benefit for bipolar disorder. There has been less study of carbamazepine's effect on second messenger systems, but it appears to reduce phosphoinositol signaling and the activities of adenylate cyclase and guanylate cyclase.

The anticonvulsant activity of lamotrigine is hypothesized to result from blockade of voltage-sensitive sodium channels, which inhibits the release of the presynaptic excitatory amino acids aspartate and glutamate. Lamotrigine also blocks high-voltage activated N- and P-type calcium channels and inhibits serotonin reuptake. To date, the influence of lamotrigine on intracellular signaling cascades is unknown.

### ANTIPSYCHOTICS

The pharmacology of antipsychotic drugs is described in Chapter 1. Their mechanism of action in the treatment of bipolar disorder is uncertain but may involve the same effects on serotonin and dopamine systems that are believed to underlie the effectiveness of these medications for schizophrenia. Atypical antipsychotics are preferred to older agents due to a reduced risk of tardive dyskinesia, a generally more benign side effect profile, and evidence of some efficacy in the treatment of bipolar depression.

## Pharmacokinetics

The pharmacokinetic properties of mood stabilizers are summarized in Table 3-2.

■ **TABLE 3-2.** Pharmacokinetics

| GENERIC NAME | TRADE NAME | PEAK PLASMA LEVELS (h) | HALF-LIFE (h) |
|---|---|---|---|
| Carbamazepine | Tegretol and others | 1.5–6 | 25–65 or 8–29 |
| Gabapentin | Neurontin | 3 | 5–7 |
| Lamotrigine | Lamictal | 1–5 | 26 |
| Lithium | Eskalith and others | 1–4 | 18–36 |
| Topiramate | Topamax | 2 | 21 |
| Valproate | Depakote and others | 2–4 | 9–16 |
| Aripiprazole | Ability | 3–5 | 75* |
| Olanzapine | Zyprexa | 6 | 27 |
| Quetiapine | Seroquel | 1.5 | 7 |
| Risperidone | Risperdal | 1 | 3** |
| Ziprasidone | Geodon | 6–8 | 4–10 |

* $t_{1/2}$ of active metabolite is 94 hours.
** $t_{1/2}$ of active metabolite is 24 hours.

## LITHIUM

Lithium is available as both immediate release lithium carbonate as well as in two slow-release formulations. The latter are generally better tolerated, produce lower peak levels for a given area under the curve, and allow for once daily administration. In any form, lithium has the following properties:

- Rapid and complete absorption after oral administration.
- Low protein binding.
- Absence of liver metabolism.
- Peak plasma levels achieved within 1.5 to 2 hours for standard preparations or 4 to 4.5 hours for slow-release forms.
- Plasma half-life of 17 to 36 hours.
- 95% drug excretion by the kidneys, with excretion proportionate to plasma concentrations.

Because lithium is filtered through the proximal tubules, factors that decrease glomerular filtration rates will decrease lithium clearance. Sodium also is filtered through the proximal tubules, so a decrease in plasma sodium can increase lithium reabsorption and lead to increased plasma lithium levels. Conversely, an increase in plasma lithium levels can cause an increase in sodium excretion, depleting plasma sodium.

### ANTICONVULSANTS

Valproate is available as valproic acid or divalproex sodium, a compound containing equal parts valproic acid and sodium valproate. Divalproex is better tolerated than valproic acid, has been studied more extensively, and is more frequently used. Divalproex is available in immediate, delayed, and extended release forms. Valproate is characterized by the following:

- Rapid absorbtion after oral administration, reaching peak plasma levels within 2 to 4 hours of ingestion.
- Bioavailability unaffected by food, though absorption may be delayed.
- Rapid distribution and high (90%) plasma protein binding.
- Half-life between 9 and 16 hours, with 1 to 4 days needed to attain steady state.

Carbamazepine is available in an immediate release and three extended release forms. It is metabolized by the hepatic cytochrome P450 2D6 system, which it also robustly induces. As a result of this *autoinduction*, the rate of metabolism of carbamazepine (and other P450 substrates) usually increases over the first several weeks of treatment (see 'Drug Interactions' on page 119). Initial steady state may be attained within 4 to 5 days, but autoinduction may delay final steady state until 3 to 4 weeks after treatment initiation. This calls for added vigilance on the part of the clinician, as the level of carbamazepine must be monitored and its dose often must be raised during this early phase of treatment. Additional pharmacokinetic properties of carbamazepine include:

- Occurrence of peak plasma levels within 4 to 6 hours after ingestion of the solid dosage form.
- Bioavailability of 85%, which may be reduced when the drug is taken with meals.
- Plasma protein binding of 80%.
- A half-life (after 3–4 weeks of treatment) ranging from 5 to 26 hours.
- Production of an active metabolite, 10, 11-epoxide, which has a half-life of about 6 hours. This metabolite, also known as oxcarbazepine, has been utilized as an anticonvulsant itself, and is undergoing clinical testing as a mood stabilizer.

Lamotrigine is primarily metabolized by glucuronic acid conjugation. Enzyme induces, such as carbamazepine, increase lamotrigine metabolism whereas competitors, such as valproate, markedly decrease its metabolism (see 'Drug Interactions' on page 119). Other pharmacokinetic parameters include:

- Complete absorbtion after oral administration.
- Bioavailability of 98%, which is unaffected by food.
- Peak plasma concentrations occurring between 1 and 2 hours after administration, but delayed to up to 5 hours in patients also taking valproate.
- Protein binding of approximately 55%, making clinically significant interactions with other protein-bound drugs unlikely.
- Half-life of 12–27 hours, increasing to 59 hours in patients also taking valproate.
- Occurrence of steady-state levels in 3 to 10 days.

**ANTIPSYCHOTICS**

The pharmacokinetic characteristics of atypical antipsychotics are described in Chapter 1.

## INDICATIONS

The principle indications in the treatment of bipolar disorder are:

- Acute mania and mixed mania
- Acute depression
- Maintenance therapy
- Rapid cycling

## DRUG SELECTION AND INITIATION OF TREATMENT

### Acute Mania

The goal of treatment should be to suppress completely all symptoms of mania and return the patient to his or her mental status *quo ante*. Mood, thinking, and behavior should normalize, though different symptom clusters may improve at different rates. For economic or social reasons, it is sometimes necessary to discharge inpatients with partially remitted mania or hypomania. In this setting, it is imperative to follow such patients closely (perhaps using partial hospitalization or intensive outpatient programs) until total remission of symptoms has occurred. In particular, it is important to monitor, and perhaps provide prophylactic pharmacotherapy, for the rapid slide into acute depression that frequently follows mania.

### Drug Selection

#### LITHIUM

For many patients with hypomania, lithium by itself can induce a total remission. Even in acute mania, response rates in clinical trials using lithium monotherapy can be as high 80–90%. In everyday clinical practice, however, the use of additional mood stabilizers (anticonvulsants or atypical antipsychotics) may be necessary for remission. In addition, manic psychosis calls for the use of adjunctive antipsychotics and in many patients use of benzodiazepines may be very helpful for symptomatic treatment of agitation and anxiety. Certain clinical features are somewhat predictive of lower lithium response rates. These include:

- Rapid cycling course
- Mixed mania
- Greater number of cumulative episodes (> 10 lifetime)
- Comorbid anxiety disorders
- Comorbid substance abuse

**ANTICONVULSANTS**
Experts usually rank lithium as the treatment of choice for a patient with classic mania, but divalproex is an acceptable first-line alternative. It may be used singly in patients who cannot tolerate lithium. For patients who do not respond to lithium, there are no secure data on whether divalproex should be added as an adjunct or substituted, but many psychiatrists would choose the former in a patient who appears to respond at least partially to lithium and the latter in patients for whom lithium seems to afford no benefit. Carbamazepine has also been used in bipolar patients non-responsive to or intolerant of lithium. This use is based upon studies using active comparators (including lithium) and demonstrating comparable overall efficacy. Despite being used for decades in this way, it is only recently that FDA approval was sought and obtained for an acute antimanic indication for a slow release form of carbamazepine. Older long prospective studies comparing carbamazepine to lithium suggested a superiority of the anticonvulsant in patients with mixed or dysphoric mania, rapid cycling, or significant comordity. As such, it appears to share a similar profile to divalproex. However, it has a rather different side effect profile, having less risk of weight gain, tremor, or hair loss, but greater risk of neurological side effects, such as ataxia, vertigo, and diplopia. Two other liabilities associated with carbamazepine include an increased risk of agranulocytosis and a robust induction of hepatic enzymes. The latter often results in more frequent blood level monitor and the need to compensate for dropping carbamazepine levels. In addition, the dosing of other medications must often be adjusted after addition of carbamazepine.

**ATYPICAL ANTIPSYCHOTICS**

With the exception of clozapine, all other atypical antipsy-chotic drugs have received approval by the FDA for use as monotherapy treatments for acute mania. Clozapine has been shown to be effective in patients with treatment-resistant symptoms but other atypicals with fewer serious adverse effects are preferred for routine use. Placebo-controlled monotherapy trials have demonstrated efficacy for olanza-pine at 10 or 15 mg/day, risperidone at 3–6 mg/day, quetiapine at 600 mg/day, ziprasidone at mean doses of either 112 or 130 mg/day, and aripiprazole at 10–15 mg/day. The presence or absence of psychosis has not been shown to influence antipsy-chotic efficacy in mania.

# Relative Efficacy of Different Agents

There are relatively few head to head comparisons of antimanic agents and the results can be summarized as follows:

- Olanzapine and valproate have been compared in two double blind studies, which yielded equivalent efficacy in one study and a modest superiority of olanzapine in the other. Tolerability favored valproate in both studies.
- Valproate and carbamazepine may have greater efficacy than lithium in patients with mixed mania, rapid cycling, or high levels of comorbidity.
- Quetiapine has performed comparably to lithium in controlled trials.
- Risperidone, quetiapine, and aripiprazole have all performed similarly to haloperidol in active comparator trials.

Acute mania is often a clinic emergency and is generally treated in an inpatient setting. Rapid mood stabilization and the reduction of agitation take priority over concerns about medication side effects. Polypharmacy is the rule in this setting, with atypical antipsychotic agents frequently added to lithium or an anticonvulsant. In support of this approach, recent studies have demonstrated improved antimanic response with the addition to lithium or valproate of olanzapine, risperidone, or quetiapine. Generally, these combinations are quite safe, but caution should be used if combining lithium with older antipsychotics as it may increase the risk of extrapyramidal effects and possibly, of neurotoxicity. In addition, the combination of thioridazine and lithium is contraindicated due to an increased risk of ventricular arrhythmias.

The American Psychiatric Association guidelines for bipolar disorder have recommend lithium or valproate plus an atypical antipsychotic as the first-line therapy for acute mania. Less severely ill patients may be treated with a single antimanic agent (lithium, valproate, or an atypical antipsychotic; this recommendation was published prior to the FDA approval of extended release carbamazepine). The Expert Consensus Guideline Series published in 2004 provides similar first-line recommendations but also lists lithium alone as a first-line treatment for euphoric mania or for non-rapid cycling hypomania. Valproate is preferred to lithium if either psychosis or rapid cycling is present. Short-term adjunctive treatment with a benzodiazepine is endorsed as an augmentation for agitation and anxiety, and for providing needed sedation. If an antidepressant appears to be linked to switching or cycle acceleration in a manic patient, it should be tapered and discontinued. Bear in mind, however, that manic episodes are often followed by a period of severe depression, and also that abrupt antidepressant discontinuation may increase the risk of a sudden manic shift. The options for treatment of acute mania are listed in Table 3-3.

### ANXIOLYTICS

Among current anxiolytic agents, benzodiazepines are usually selected as adjuncts to treat acute mania because of their safety and efficacy. Although some have claimed specific antimanic efficacy for clonazepam or other benzodiazepines, most psychiatrists are more impressed with their benefits as adjunctive sedatives than with more specific antimanic activity. Lorazepam is often the benzodiazepine selected for this indication because it yields predictable blood levels when administered intramuscularly. Benzodiazepines have a wide margin of safety and can be safely administered in even very high doses, suppressing potentially dangerous excitement and allowing patients much needed sleep. When used together with an antipsychotic agent, benzodiazepines counteract the

■ **TABLE 3-3.** Treatments for Acute Mania

| TREATMENT | ADVANTAGES | DISADVANTAGES |
|---|---|---|
| Lithium | Efficacy: 70–80% | Side effects: sedation, weight gain, tremor hair loss, polyuria Low therapeutic index |
| Valproate | Comparable efficacy to Li May be better in mixed states | Side effects: sedation, weight gain, tremor, hair loss |
| Carbamazepine | Comparable efficacy to Li May be better in mixed states | Side effects: neurologic (ataxia, vertigo, diplopia) |
| Atypical Antipsychotics | Comparable efficacy to Li | Side effects, differ by individual agent. Risk of tardive dyskinesia |
| Typical Antipsychotics | Comparable efficacy to Li Rapid onset of action | May worsen bipolar depression. Greater risk of tardive dyskinesia |
| Electroconvulsive Therapy | Efficacy ~80%. Safe for patients unable to take medication | More difficult to administer. Long-term effectiveness unclear |
| Anxiolytics | Good as adjunctive sedatives, wide margin of safety | Probably not specifically antimanic. Potential abuse and dependence |

antipsychotic agent's tendency to provoke extrapyramidal reactions and seizures. For lorazepam, 1 to 2 mg can be administered by mouth or intramuscularly as frequently as hourly.

## Treatment Initiation and Dose Titration

It is important to carry out a range of tests before embarking on treatment to identify patients at increased risk of adverse effects (Table 3-4).

### LITHIUM
Pretreatment testing for lithium includes a complete blood count, electrolyte determinations, renal panel, and thyroid function tests. An electrocardiogram should also be obtained.

■ **TABLE 3-4.** Pretreatment Tests

| MEDICATION | TESTING |
| --- | --- |
| Any Medication | • Comprehensive medical history |
| | • Physical examination including vital signs and weight |
| | • Pregnancy test, if applicable |
| Lithium | • Complete blood count |
| | • Electrolytes |
| | • Renal panel (blood urea nitrogen, creatinine, and routine urinalysis) |
| | • Thyroid panel plus thyroid-stimulating hormone |
| | • Electrocardiogram |
| Valproate | • Complete blood count |
| | • Liver function tests |
| Carbamazepine | • Complete blood count |
| | • Liver function tests |
| | • Renal panel |
| | • Urinalysis |
| Atypical Antipsychotics | • Blood glucose |
| | • Blood lipids |

Lithium dosage may be based on a plasma concentration sampled 12 hours after the last dose, or the drug may be gradually titrated to a dose that is tolerated and within the range usually considered "therapeutic." As with any drug, approximately five half-lives must elapse for steady state to be achieved; for an average adult, this takes about five days for lithium (longer in the elderly or in patients with impaired renal function). To treat acute mania, plasma concentrations should typically be greater than 0.8 mEq/L but to avoid toxicity the level should not exceed 1.5 mEq/L. It is important to know what other medications a patient may be taking because many drugs interact with lithium and can lead to increased or decreased lithium levels and possibly to adverse effects (see 'Drug Interactions' on page 119).

To reach therapeutic levels rapidly in healthy younger patients with normal renal and cardiac function, the psychiatrist may prescribe 300 mg of lithium carbonate four times daily from the outset, sampling the first plasma level after five days (or sooner should toxic signs become apparent). Thereafter, the dose should be adjusted to achieve a 12-hour plasma concentration between 0.8 and 1.3 mEq/L at steady state. By contrast, in a patient with mild hypomanic symptoms it may be wiser to begin with a lower lithium dose, such as 300 mg b.i.d., taking longer to achieve therapeutic levels but minimizing side effects that could trouble the patient and promote medication non-adherence. Once steady state has been achieved at therapeutic concentrations and the patient is clinically stable, lithium can be administered to most patients in a once-daily dose, usually at bedtime. Not only is this schedule easier to remember, but it tends to decrease such common side effects as tremor and polyuria.

### ANTICONVULSANTS
Before initiating treatment with valproate or divalproex, the psychiatrist should obtain a comprehensive medical history and ensure that a physical examination has been performed, with particular attention to suggestions of liver disease or bleeding abnormalities (see Table 3-4). Baseline liver and hematological functions are measured before treatment, every one to four weeks for the first six months, and then once every three to six months. Mild elevations in transaminase levels are not uncommon and should be monitored, but tend to be mild and self-limited, not requiring discontinuation of the medication. Evidence of abnormalities in hemostasis or coagulation, such as hemorrhage or increased bruising, should prompt a reduction of dosage or withdrawal of therapy. The drug should be discontinued immediately in the presence of significant hepatic dysfunction.

In healthy adults, divalproex is started at 750 mg/day in divided doses and then adjusted to achieve a 12-hour serum valproate concentration between 50 and 125 μg/mL. The time of dosing is determined by possible side effects (particularly sedation), and once-a-day dosing can be employed if tolerated. The use of slow-release formulations reduces side effects (particularly gastrointestinal) and facilitates the use of once daily dosing. As with lithium, the antimanic response to valproate typically occurs after one to two weeks. It may be possible to obtain a faster response with oral loading of divalproex at 20 mg/kg/day for the first five days. This produces serum concentrations greater than 50 mg/L after two days of treatment and is generally well tolerated with few side effects.

Carbamazepine is typically started at 200 to 400 mg/day in three or four divided doses, and increased to 800 to 1000 mg/day by the end of the first week. As with divalproex, slow release formulations may improve tolerability and facilitate use of once daily dosing. If clinical improvement is insufficient by the end of the second week, and the patient has not had intolerable side effects to the drug, carbamazepine may be increased to as high as 1600 mg/day. As there is little data relating carbamazepine blood levels and psychiatric efficacy, the anti-epileptic blood level range (4 to 15 ng/mL) is generally utilized. If carbamazepine is combined with lithium or antipsychotics, lower doses and blood levels of carbamazepine may suffice. If divalproex and carbamazepine are administered simultaneously, blood levels of each should be monitored carefully because of the complex pharmacokinetic interactions between the two agents.

**ANTIPSYCHOTICS**

Although in the 1970s it was commonplace to use ultra-high doses of antipsychotics in attempts to suppress psychotic symptoms (sometimes in excess of 100 mg of haloperidol daily), this is seldom necessary and may be counterproductive: it can increase the risk of acute cardiovascular complications, seizures, acute dystonia, and possibly neuroleptic malignant syndrome. However, in emergent situations, intramuscular (IM) administration of an antipsychotic can help reduce agitation more rapidly than lithium or an anticonvulsant. IM formulations exist for several first-generation antipsychotics and but only for one atypical antipsychotics, ziprasidone.

Dosing recommendations for atypical antipsychotics are listed in Table 3-5.

Recently, significant concern has been raised about the risks of metabolic complications associated with the use of atypical antipsychotics. Weight gain, hyperlipidemia, and diabetes (including abrupt and often catastrophic new onset diabetes) have been observed to occur at relatively high rates. Although the FDA has mandated a black box warning for

■ **TABLE 3-5.** Atypicals in the Treatment of Acute Mania

| GENERIC NAME | BRAND NAME | DOSE ON FIRST DAY | ACUTE DOSE ADJUSTMENT | MAINTENANCE DOSE |
|---|---|---|---|---|
| Aripiprazole | Ability | 15–30 mg *q.i.d.* | – | 15–30 mg *q.i.d.* |
| Olanzapine | Zyprexa | 10–15 *q.i.d.* | increments of 5 mg per day | 5–20 mg *q.i.d.* |
| Quetiapine | Seroquel | 50 mg *b.i.d.* | 200 mg *b.i.d.* by day 4 in increments of 50 mg *b.i.d.* | 200–400 mg *b.i.d.* |
| Risperidone | Risperdal | 2–3 mg *q.i.d.* | increments of 1 mg per day | 1–6 mg *q.i.d.* |
| Ziprasidone | Geodon (po) | 40 mg *b.i.d.* | 60–80 mg *b.i.d.* on day 2 | 40–80 mg *b.i.d.* |
|  | Geodon (im) | 10 mg q2hr |  |  |

the entire class of atypical antipsychotics, the risk does appear to be greatest with clozapine and olanzapine. The Consensus Development Conference on Antipsychotic Drugs and Obesity and Diabetes has made recommendations for screening prior to treatment with an atypical antipsychotic and for monitoring during treatment. Before starting the medication, weigh potential benefits against metabolic and medical risks based upon the following assessments:

• Personal and family history of diabetes, obesity, hyperlipidemia, hypertension, and cardiovascular disease
• Baseline height and weight (which should be used to calculate the body mass index, BMI) and waist circumference (measured at the height of the umbilicus)
• Blood pressure
• Fasting plasma glucose
• Fasting lipid profile

The presence of metabolic abnormalities or significant personal or family history might prompt preferential use of atypical antipsychotics with lower risk (ziprasidone or aripiprazole) or intermediate risk (risperidone or quetiapine) relative to higher risk (olanzapine and clozapine).

Follow up monitoring of patients on atypical antipsychotics should be conducted as follows:

- Review personal and family history annually.
- Measure weight and BMI at 4, 8, and 12 weeks, then quarterly.
- Measure waist circumference annually.
- Measure blood pressure and fasting plasma glucose at 12 weeks, then annually.
- Measure fasting lipids at 12 weeks, then every five years.

## Acute Depression

Long-term prospective studies have demonstrated that depression is much more frequent and protracted than mood elevation in bipolar disorder, particularly for bipolar II disorder, and accounts for a much greater proportion of time spent ill. The depressed phase of bipolar illness is also the phase most associated with suicide attempts and residual depressive symptoms are most predictive of functional impairments in partially remitted bipolar patients. Unfortunately, depression occurring in bipolar disorder is also the syndrome of the illness for which we have the least effective and safe treatments. Traditional antidepressants often promote increased mood instability, cycle acceleration, and mood switching from depression to mania or hypomania. Tricyclic antidepressants are the most likely to trigger instability, but no antidepressant has been shown to be completely safe in this regard. In light of this fact, as well as the robust antidepressant effects of some newer mood stabilizers, traditional antidepressants should not be the first-line treatment for bipolar depression. Treatments for acute depression in bipolar disorder are shown in Table 3-6.

## Drug Selection

Current guidelines by the American Psychiatric Association list lithium or lamotrigine as first-line monotherapy for acute bipolar depression. Antidepressant monotherapy is not recommended except in combination with lithium in severely ill patients. The recommendation for lamotrigine use as a first-line treatment derives from two sources. The first is a large double

■ **TABLE 3-6.** Treatments for Acute Depression in Bipolar Disorder

| TREATMENT | ADVANTAGES | DISADVANTAGES |
| --- | --- | --- |
| Mood stabilizers | Provide maintenance and antimanic efficacy | Antidepressant efficacy relatively modest for most mood stabilizers |
| | If use of antidepressants becomes necessary, should reduce the risk of switching or cycle acceleration | Side effects may be problematic: sedation, weight gain/metabolic, tremor, etc. |
| Lamotrigine | Significantly more efficacious than most other mood stabilizers. | Antimanic efficacy is relatively modest, so may not provide comprehensive treatment as monotherapy for bipolar I patients |
| | No evidence of induction of switching or rapid cycling | |
| | Generally well tolerated | |
| Quetiapine | Recent data suggest comparable efficacy to lamotrigine | Side effects may be problematic: sedation, weight gain/metabolic |
| | May be efficacious for depression at doses lower than those require for mania, improving tolerability | Risk of tardive dyskinesia with long-term treatment |
| | At higher doses may be able to provide balanced and strong antidepressant and antimanic efficacy | |
| Antidepressants | Probably efficacious in the acute setting | Can trigger switch into mania and increase cycling |
| ECT | Acutely efficacious | Cognitive side effects |
| | Safe for patients unable to take medication (e.g., pregnancy) | Need for anesthesia |
| | | Maintenance after acute treatment problematic |

blind, placebo controlled trial of lamotrigine monotherapy (50 mg vs. 200 mg final dose, after appropriate titration). The response rate with the 200 mg final dose was 56%, which was significantly greater than that of placebo using several clinical measures. Though the study was not powered to fully test this, the results of the study suggested that the 200 mg final dose was more effective than 50 mg final dose. The second line of evidence supporting lamotrigine for bipolar depression comes from a larger prospective maintenance study of remitted bipolar I and II patients, comparing lamotrigine monotherapy at 200 mg with lithium monotherapy and with placebo. In this study, lamotrigine was superior to placebo for prophylaxis of depressive or elevated relapses, but more robustly so for depression. In contrast, lithium was more effective in prevented elevation. Furthermore, unlike with traditional antidepressants, there is no clear evidence of lamotrigine provoking cycling or switching.

Recently, quetiapine has emerged as a second mood stabilizer with potentially robust antidepressant efficacy. A large multicenter placebo controlled study (There are 2 studies: BOLDER studies) compared quetiapine monotherapy at two doses (300 mg and 600 mg) in bipolar I and II patients in an acute major depression. Response and remission rates for both active groups were identical (58% and 36%, respectively) and significantly better than for the placebo group. The effect size for quetiapine in this study was comparable to that of lamotrigine for bipolar depression and significantly greater than that of olanzapine when used as a monotherapy for bipolar depression.

Apart from lamotrigine and quetiapine, there are few data available to stratify the other mood stabilizers in terms of antidepressant efficacy. Lithium, carbamazepine, and olanzapine appear to be effective for bipolar depression at a much lower rate than lamotrigine or quetiapine, and risperidone, ziprasidone, and aripiprazole have insufficient data to evaluate. Nevertheless, there is reason to consider lithium seriously in patients with persistent, frequent, or severe bipolar depression. Lithium is the only pharmacologic intervention that exhibits a specific anti-suicide effect, to some degree independent of its mood efficacy within patients. Lithium treatment reduces the suicide rate in bipolar patients approximately seven-fold. However, in the same samples, discontinuation of lithium results in a rapid return to previous (or even, transiently, to higher) suicide rates. Moreover, when tapered quickly or abruptly discontinued, a twenty-fold increase in suicides and attempts occurs in the first year. Comparable anti-suicide efficacy in bipolar patients has not been demonstrated for anti-convulsants or antipsychotics, though confirmation of lithium's uniqueness will require more studies of other agents. In addition, both lithium and anticonvulsants can have a positive impact on impulsivity and aggression, two important suicide risk factors.

Probably all available antidepressant drugs can be effective in treating bipolar depression but we lack sufficient data to stratify them in terms of efficacy. There is some evidence that MAO inhibitors may be somewhat more effective than other classes but they may also be more likely than other classes of antidepressants (except for TCAs) to provoke mood instability. Of course, antidpressants should never be prescribed for bipolar patients in the absence of adequate mood stabilizers, which reduce the risk of switching or cycle acceleration. If mania occurs, the antidepressant medication should be discontinued immediately. It is not clear how long antidepressants should be continued following resolution of an acute major depression. The Expert Consensus Guidelines recommended continuing antidepressants for 18–30 weeks in non-rapid cycling bipolar I patients following resolution of depression and for 9–17 weeks in rapid cycling patients.

## Treatment Initiation and Dose Titration

Dosing guideline for lithium should parallel those for hypo-manic patients, trading slower titration and the risk of delayed response to minimize side effects and risk of toxicity. However, the target blood level should still be set at 0.8 or greater. Dosing guidelines for lamotrigine are particularly important to follow, as a more accelerated rate of titration significantly increases the risk of Stevens-Johnson Syndrome (SJS), an immune-mediated systemic reaction which often present with a severe rash and

■ **TABLE 3-7.** Lamotrigine Dosing

|  | NO ANTICONVULSANTS | WITH VALPROATE | WITH CBZ |
|---|---|---|---|
| Weeks 1 & 2 | 25 mg/d | 12.5 mg/d | 50 mg/d |
| Weeks 3 & 4 | 50 mg/d | 25 mg/d | 50 mg b.i.d. |
| Week 5+ | Add 50–100 mg every 1–2 weeks | Add 25–50 mg every 1–2 weeks | Add 100 mg/d every 1–2 weeks |
| Maintenance | 100–400 mg | 100–200 mg/d | 250 mg b.i.d. |

has a 10–15% mortality rate (see 'Adverse Effects' on page 111). The dosing of lamotrigine is also complicated by pharmacokinetic interactions (Table 3-7). Specifically, clearance of lamotrigine is reduced by valproate, causing an approximate doubling of blood levels for a given dose and requiring, therefore, that doses at each point in the titration be halved compared to the lamotrigine monotherapy titration. Conversely, lamotrigine levels are cut roughly in half by P450 enzyme inducing medications such as carbamazepine. This permits an increase in the dose at any point in the titration compared to monotherapy dosing.

Quetiapine dosing for depression can proceed more slowly than for mania. Since 300 mg was identical in efficacy to 600 mg in the primary study (two Studies – BOLDER I and BOLDER II) informing the use of quetiapine for depression, it is prudent to have a lower target dose and provide sufficient time during the titration to allow for responses at lower doses. A slower titration and lower target might also reduce side effects and the potential for metabolic complications.

## Breakthrough Episodes

The first step in managing a breakthrough episode of either mania or depression is to check medication adherence, evaluate other potential precipitants of relapse (e.g., seasonal changes, which are common in bipolar disorder, onset of perimenopause, severe stressors, recurrent substance abuse, etc.) and evaluate medication doses and blood levels. Patients on lithium should have thyroid function tests checked as well, since hypothyroidism secondary to lithium treatment can destabilize mood. Some data also suggest that levels of free T4 in the euthyroid but low normal range prolong episodes of bipolar depression and reduce the likelihood of successful treatment.

In parallel with addressing any clear precipitants, the medication regimen must be thoughtfully and deliberately adjusted to both provide treatment for the acute episode and also to improve the level of prophylactic efficacy. Primary mood stabilizer doses should be increased as tolerated, particularly for relapse into elevation, and use of additional medications considered (e.g., adding lamotrigine for relapse into depression). If a pattern of increased mood instability and increased cycling becomes apparent, then serious consideration should be given to discontinuing any antidepressant in the regimen, even if the most recent relapse was into a depressed state. Often the best treatment for rapid cycling is not the addition of any medication but the discontinuation of an antidepressant. Consistent use by the patient of a daily prospective mood rating instrument, such as the Life Chart, can be very helpful for discerning an increase in instability.

## Maintenance

Nowhere is the potential gap between the results of clinical trials and clinical experience more apparent than in maintenance treatment. For example, valproate is one of the most commonly used maintenance treatments for bipolar disorder and most psychiatrists agree that it is clearly quite effective in this role. The Expert Consensus Guidelines also endorse valproate as a first-line maintenance treatment. This is true despite the absence of a large scale study clearly demonstrating this robust effect. Fortunately recent years have witnessed a significant increase in maintenance studies and some of these data can now inform treatment selection.

The risk of relapse is particularly high in the six months following an acute episode. Psychosocial interventions should be offered in addition to drug treatments, which are summarized in Table 3-8.

■ **TABLE 3-8.** Advantages and Disadvantages of Specific Maintenance Treatments.

| TREATMENT | ADVANTAGES | DISADVANTAGES |
|---|---|---|
| Lithium | Most robust dataset and clearly very effective for prevention of mania | Side effects and low therapeutic index |
| | Specific anti-suicide effect | Lethality in overdose |
| | | Risk of renal damage |
| Valproate | Possibly comparable to lithium | Weight gain and other side effects |
| | May be more effective for patients with rapid cycling, mixed episodes and comorbidity | Teratogenicity, for female patients in reproductive years |
| Olanzapine | Possibly comparable to lithium for prevention of mania | Weight gain and metabolic risks |
| | | Tardive dyskinesia risk |
| Lamotrigine | Probably more effective than other mood stabilizers for depression | Probably somewhat less effective for prevention of mania |
| | Generally better tolerated than other mood stabilizers | |
| Carbamazepine | Profile comparable to valproate | More maintenance data needed |
| | Less risk of weight gain | |
| Typical antipsychotics | Likely good for prophylaxis of mania | May worsen depression |
| | | High risk of tardive dyskinesia |
| Antidepressants | May prevent recurrence of depression | May precipitate mania and provoke rapid cycling |
| ECT | Acutely effective for both mania and depression | Not adequately studied |
| | | Maintenance of acute response may be poor |
| Psychotherapy | As adjunct, increases medication compliance, overall functioning | Not efficacious alone |

## LITHIUM

For bipolar maintenance, lithium has the longest and largest database of clinical experience and by far the greatest number of patients studied in rigorous clinical trials. In randomized trials, the relapse rate in patients treated with lithium is about 37% compared with 79% with placebo. Predictors of poor response to lithium are listed in Table 3-9.

Most patients starting lithium maintenance are already taking lithium after an acute episode. A medical history should also have been obtained that included questions about: past medical and family history of renal, thyroid, cardiac, and central nervous system disorders; other drugs a patient may be taking (including prescription, over-the-counter, and illicit); the use of such common substances as caffeine, nicotine, and alcohol; and special diets or diet supplements. They should also have had baseline medical tests, including assessment of thyroid function (thyroid panel plus thyroid-stimulating hormone) and renal function (blood urea nitrogen, creatinine, and routine urinalysis), a complete blood count, electrolyte determinations, an electrocardiogram, and a physical examination (see Table 3-4).

If a patient who is to start lithium maintenance therapy is not already taking lithium, a slower titration than that used for acute mania can be utilized. A physically healthy, average-size adult may be started with 300 mg of lithium carbonate twice daily, or 600 mg at night if a slow release formulation is employed. An elderly, ill, or slightly built individual can begin with as little as 300 mg per day. Because it takes about five days

■ **TABLE 3-9.** Predictors of Poor Response to Lithium Prophylaxis

Rapid or continuous cycling
Mixed states or dysphoric mania
Alcohol or drug abuse
Non-compliance with treatment
Cycle pattern of depression–mania–euthymia
Personality disturbance
History of poor interepisode functioning
Poor social support system
Three or more prior episodes

to achieve a steady state (longer in the elderly and those with renal impairment), a 12 hour trough lithium level should be drawn at approximately that interval. Dose adjustments can be made at intervals of five or more days, with repeat levels as needed to obtain a therapeutic level. Levels between 0.8 and 1.0 mEq/L afford threefold greater protection against recurrent episodes than a range of 0.4 to 0.6 mEq/L. Furthermore, patients in the higher range are less likely to experience subsyndromal symptoms (hypomania or minor depression) and, if such symptoms do appear, are less likely to go on to a full episode. However, higher blood levels are associated with more side effects and the risk of non-compliance. Sometimes education and reassurance are sufficient to keep patients at higher levels. In addition, remedies are available to treat some of the more aggravating side effects (e.g., beta blockers for tremor). Side effects may diminish with a decrease in lithium level, but both psychiatrist and patient should be aware that this may decrease the level of protection against mood swings.

There have been no systematic studies of the lithium level–clinical response relationship in elderly patients, but because older people are more sensitive to side effects, it may be prudent to attempt to maintain elderly bipolar patients at lower plasma lithium concentrations. It should also be kept in mind that a given dose will frequently produce higher blood levels as a person ages (likely due to gradual reduction in renal function), so dose reduction may be necessary over time.

Monitoring of patients on maintenance lithium treatment focuses on three elements: blood level, renal function, and thyroid function. The following is a reasonable regimen for monitoring over time:

- Lithium level every 3 months.
- Electrolytes, blood urea nitrogen, and creatinine every six months, or sooner if the lithium level rises acutely and without any other explanation.
- TSH, and free and total T4 every six months, or sooner if the patient's mood becomes more unstable or symptoms suggestive of hypothyroidism occur.
- An annual electrocardiogram for men over 40 and women over 50 years of age.

If lithium needs to be discontinued for any reason, it is preferable to taper the medication over six or more weeks. Rapid discontinuation increases the risk of relapse and may further increase the risk of suicidal actions.

It can be very difficult to determine whether a symptom, such as a minor drop in mood or several days of reduced sleep, represents a transient fluctuation or is a harbinger of a major affective episode. Daily mood charting and close contact with patient can help in this determination and also provide the opportunity to rapidly respond to an incipient relapse. Mild hypomanic symptoms may be more likely to be predictive of a manic relapse than depressive symptoms predictive of a recurrence of major depression. As described above, optimizing current medications and adding adjunctive treatments (e.g., benzodiazepine in a patient who feels slightly agitated and is not sleeping well) may be sufficient to prevent a more dramatic worsening in mood.

### ANTICONVULSANTS

Valproate is an important alternative to lithium as a maintenance treatment for bipolar disorder. It may be preferable for patients with rapid cycling, a history of dysphoric or mixed mania, comorbid substance abuse or anxiety disorders, or organic brain disease. Carbamazepine has a somewhat greater medical risk, in terms of bone marrow suppression, but may be better tolerated than valproate for some patients. In clinical trials, approximately 60% of patients have a moderate or marked response to carbamazepine compared with 22% with placebo. In comparisons with lithium, carbamazepine was associated with equivalent or greater rates of improvement. Although no head to head comparisons exist for valproate and carbamazepine in maintenance treatment, other clinical data and experience suggest that they are comparably effective and work well in an overlapping subset of patients.

When valproate is used for maintenance therapy, it is best to start with a low dose, such as 250 to 500 mg daily, building the dose gradually to maintain a plasma level between 50 and 125 μg/mL. Treatment with carbamazepine should be initiated at a low dose, 100 mg/day, increasing in increments of

100 mg/day every four to five days. Dosing is usually two to four times daily for the immediate release formulations. Although a correlation between blood level and clinical response has yet to be established, most psychiatrists are guided by the therapeutic range in patients with epilepsy: usually 4 to 15 μg/mL. Most patients taking carbamazepine for bipolar disorder are maintained with doses between 400 and 1800 mg/day. Because of enzyme induction, it is often necessary to increase the dose after two to three weeks of treatment to maintain the same blood level.

As described above, in the section on treatment of bipolar depression, two large maintenance trials evaluated lamotrigine relative to lithium and placebo in remitted bipolar I and II patients. Lamotrigine was more robust in preventing relapse into depression and lithium was more robust in preventing relapse into mania, but both agents has some, albeit lower, efficacy in preventing the other phase (i.e., lithium for depression and lamotrigine for mania). As a broad maintenance regimen, it is certainly worth considering combining a predominantly antidepressant mood stabilizer, such as lamotrigine with a predominantly antimanic one, such as lithium.

## ANTIPSYCHOTICS

More data are gradually emerging to support the efficacy of atypical antipsychotics as maintenance treatments for bipolar disorder. Olanzapine has the largest dataset to date and appears to have a profile similar to lithium, valproate, and carbamazepine, being more effective for prevention of mania than for prevention of depression. It is too early to judge the other atypical antipsychotics in terms of relative efficacy for prevention of mania and depression.

One major drawback to the use of atypical antipsychotics for maintenance is the cumulative risk for tardive dyskinesia. Unfortunately, at this time there are insufficient data to clearly weigh that risk or to stratify specific agents. However, assuming comparable efficacy, one might argue that lithium and the anticonvulsants should be considered ahead of atypical antipsychotics as maintenance treatments.

## Rapid Cycling

Patients with rapid-cycling bipolar disorder—defined as four or more affective episodes in one year, with or without an intervening period of euthymia—tend to be less responsive to lithium treatment. Indeed, the initial description of rapid cycling arose from studies of lithium failure during maintenance treatment. Whether rapid cycling is a natural progression of the illness or a separate disorder has yet to be determined, but there are certain risk factors for rapid cycling. Those include gender (women comprise 70% of rapid cycling patients), use of antidepressants, and current or past thyroid disease.

Apart from the reduced effectiveness of lithium in rapid cycling, there are relatively few data to guide medication selection for the treatment of rapid cycling. More data support the use of anticonvulsants in this population, but atypical antipychotics may also be superior to lithium in this setting. One important intervention to consider is discontinuation of any antidepressant medications, even in the setting of a depressive relapse. As with any breakthrough episode, rapid cycling should be approached by evaluating mood stabilizer adherence, dosage, and blood levels. Thyroid function should be checked and any hypothyroidism addressed.

## Costs

The costs of the most widely used drugs as of December 2005 are summarized in Table 3-10.

■ **TABLE 3-10.** Current medication costs. THIS IS HIGHLY VARIABLE AND EVER-CHANGING

| MEDICATION | FORMULATION | QUANTITY | PRICE ($) |
| --- | --- | --- | --- |
| Depakene | 250 mg caps | 100 | 207.01 |
| Lithium Carbonate | 150 mg caps | 100 | 15.54 |
| | 300 mg caps | 100 | 17.77 |
| | 600 mg caps | 100 | 42.30 |
| Lithium CR* | 450 mg tabs | 180 | 81.97 |
| Valproic Acid | 250 mg caps | 100 | 29.97 |

| | | | |
|---|---|---|---|
| Divalproex sodium | 125 mg EC tabs | 180 | 110.29 |
| | 250 mg EC tabs | 180 | 204.61 |
| | 500 mg EC tabs | 180 | 359.96 |
| | 250 mg 24 hr tabs | 90 | 112.84 |
| | 500 mg 24 hr tabs | 90 | 186.28 |
| Carbamazepine | 200 mg tabs | 180 | 31.99 |
| Tegretol XR | 200 mg 12 hr tabs | 180 | 118.24 |
| | 400 mg 12 hr tabs | 180 | 149.89 |
| Trileptal | 150 mg tabs | 180 | 206.96 |
| | 300 mg tabs | 180 | 343.96 |
| | 600 mg tabs | 180 | 683.48 |
| Zyprexa | 2.5 mg tab | 100 | 522.19 |
| | 5 mg tab | 100 | 616.66 |
| | 7.5 mg tab | 100 | 746.66 |
| | 10 mg tab | 100 | 955.54 |
| | 15 mg tab | 100 | 1244.43 |
| | 20 mg tab | 100 | 1717.74 |
| | 25 mg tab | 100 | 174.28 |
| Quetiapine | 100 mg tab | 100 | 295.86 |
| | 200 mg tab | 100 | 556.08 |
| | 300 mg tab | 100 | 744.58 |
| Risperidone | 0.25 mg tab | 100 | 284.42 |
| | 0.5 mg tab | 100 | 312.74 |
| | 1 mg tab | 100 | 315.52 |
| | 2 mg tab | 100 | 534.54 |
| | 3 mg tab | 100 | 555.52 |
| | 4 mg tab | 100 | 824.99 |
| Ziprasidone | 20 mg cap | 100 | 433.32 |
| | 40 mg cap | 100 | 440.31 |
| | 60 mg cap | 100 | 479.50 |
| | 80 mg cap | 100 | 498.29 |
| Ability | 5 mg tab | 100 | 974.34 |
| | 10 mg tab | 100 | 1011.15 |
| | 15 mg tab | 100 | 971.81 |
| | 20 mg tab | 100 | 1345.07 |
| | 30 mg tab | 100 | 1345.07 |

* CR = controlled release.

## ADVERSE EFFECTS

### LITHIUM

One major limitation of lithium is its narrow therapeutic index; plasma concentrations only slightly higher than the therapeutic range can have severe side effects. Levels of 2.0 mEq/L and above, particularly if prolonged, can cause central nervous system impairment, renal shutdown, coma, permanent brain injury, and death. Management of severe lithium intoxication (Table 3-11) may require hemodialysis and medical intensive care to maintain fluid and electrolyte balance, prevent further absorption of the drug, and maximize the rate of elimination.

To avoid this, patients and their families need to be instructed carefully on a number of matters related to lithium levels. They should be alerted to the early signs of intoxication—such as increased tremor, confusion, and ataxia—and directed to stop

■ **TABLE 3-11.** Management of Serious Lithium Toxicity

1. Rapidly assess (including clinical signs and symptoms, serum lithium levels, electrolytes, and electrocardiogram), monitor vital signs, and make an accurate diagnosis.
2. Discontinue lithium therapy.
3. Support vital functions and monitor cardiac status.
4. Limit absorption.

   a. If patient is alert, provide an emetic.
   b. If patient is obtunded, intubate and suction nasogastrically (prolonged suction may be helpful because lithium levels in gastric fluid may remain high for days).

5. Prevent infection in comatose patients by body rotation and pulmonary toilet.
6. When lithium has reached nontoxic levels, vigorously hydrate (ideally 5 to 6 L/d); monitor and balance the electrolytes.
7. In moderately severe cases:

   a. Implement osmotic diuresis with urea, 20 g given intravenously two to five times per day, or mannitol, 50 to 100 g/d, given intravenously.
   b. Increase lithium clearance with aminophylline, 0.5 g up to every 6 hours, and alkalinize the urine with intravenously administered sodium lactate.
   c. Ensure adequate intake of sodium chloride to promote excretion of lithium.

8. Implement hemodialysis in the most severe cases. These are characterized by:

   a. Serum lithium levels between 2 and 4 mEq/L with severe clinical signs and symptoms (particularly decreasing urinary output and deepening CNS depression).
   b. Serum lithium levels greater than 4 mEq/L.

taking further lithium and contact their psychiatrist promptly. A lithium level should be obtained as soon as possible that same day and the symptoms followed closely for the next several days. The psychiatrist should also be contacted if the patient develops new gastrointestinal symptoms, especially vomiting or diarrhea. These symptoms may reflect an elevated lithium level or may, even if caused by an unrelated factor (such as gastrointestinal infection), trigger an elevation in the lithium level as a consequence of fluid and electrolyte changes. Other causes of fluid loss with insufficient replacement, such as excessive sweating due to heat exposure or fever, should also prompt a temporary discontinuation of lithium treatment until fluid balance is restored. Concomitant use of other medications may also increase levels of lithium and lead to lithium intoxication (See 'Drug Interactions').

The most common adverse effects from lithium are (Table 3-12):

- nausea
- vomiting
- diarrhea
- postural tremor
- polydipsia
- polyuria

If troublesome, these can usually be mitigated by altering the lithium timing or formulation or by adding a remedy. Specific interventions include the following:

- Beta blocking drugs generally dramatically reduce or completely eliminate lithium tremor. Propranolol is often used and must be dosed b.i.d. or t.i.d. to cover the entire day (unless a long acting form of propranolol is used). Treatment is initiated at 10 mg b.i.d. to t.i.d. and increased as tolerated and needed. Doses above 160 mg are not usually required.
- Diuretics for polydipsia or polyuria. Diuretics may paradoxically decrease urine volume, but because some (such as thiazides) can also raise the serum lithium concentration, lithium level must be carefully monitored and the lithium dose adjusted downward appropriately. Potassium levels should also be monitored and supplementation may be necessary.

■ **TABLE 3-12.** Adverse Effects: Lithium, Valproate, and Carbamazepine

## LITHIUM

| *Common* | *Rare* | *Rare* |
|---|---|---|
| Dermatitis | Ataxia | Hyperparathyroidism |
| Fatigue | Autonomic slowing of | Hyperthyroidism |
| Gastrointestinal | bladder and bowel | Metallic taste |
| upset | function | Nystagmus |
| Headache | Cardiovascular | Organic brain |
| Hypothyroidism | complications | syndrome |
| Memory and | Diabetes mellitus | Parathyroid hyperplasia |
| concentration | Dysarthria | and parathyroid |
| difficulties | Edema | adenomas |
| Muscle weakness | Elevated WBC | Tearing, itching, |
| Polydipsia | count | burning, or blurring |
| Polyuria | Extrapyramidal | of the eyes |
| Tremor | reactions | Tinnitus |
| Weight gain | Goiter | Vertigo |
| | Hypercalcemia | Visual distortion |

## VALPROATE

| | | |
|---|---|---|
| Alopecia | Acute pancreatitis | Hepatotoxicity |
| Gastrointestinal | Anemia (including | Hypofibrinogenemia |
| upset | macrocytic with or | Hyponatremia |
| Sedation | without folate | Incoordination |
| Tremor | deficiency) | Irreguar menses |
| Weight loss | Asterixis | Leukopenia |
| Weight gain | Ataxia | Macrocytosis |
| | Bone marrow | Nystagmus |
| | suppression | Parotid gland swelling |
| | Breast enlargement | Photosensitivity |
| | Coma | Porphyria, acute |
| | Dermatitis | intermittent |
| | Diplopia, Dizziness | Pruritus |
| | Dysarthria | Relative lymphocytosis |
| | Edema of the | Secondary amenorrhea |
| | extremities | Stevens-Johnson |
| | Encephalopathy with | syndrome |
| | fever | SIADH |
| | Enuresis | Thrombocytopenia |
| | Eosinophilia, Erythema | Thyroid function test |
| | multiforme | abnormalities |
| | Galactorrhea | |
| | Hallucinations | |
| | Headache | |

**CARBAMAZEPINE**

*Common (Diminish in Time or With Temporary Reduction in Dose)*

Ataxia
Blurred vision
Diplopia
Dizziness
Drowsiness
Fatigue
Headache
Nausea

*Less Common*

Cardiovascular complications
Gastrointestinal upset
Hyponatremia
Skin reactions (if severe, may require discontinuation of carbamazepine)

*Uncommon*

Cognitive impairment
Chills
Genitourinary effects
Fever

Hepatitis
Increased intraocular pressure
Jaundice, cholestatic and hepatocellular
Liver function abnormalities
Renal damage leading to oliguria and hypertension
SIADH
Transient leukopenia (carbamazepine may be continued unless infection develops)
Water intoxication

*Rare*

Agranulocytosis
Aplastic anemia
Lupus erythematosus-like syndrome
Pulmonary hypersensitivity

---

*SIADH*, Syndrome of inappropriate secretion of antidiuretic hormone.

- Gastrointestinal problems may be alleviated by taking lithium with food or switching to a slow release preparation (particularly if gastric distress is the problem).
- Many skin reactions have been described in association with lithium therapy, including atopic dermatitis, acne, psoriasis, and hair loss. These can usually be treated by standard dermatological means but occasionally are severe enough to force the discontinuation of therapy.
- Electrocardiographic effects of lithium are also usually benign and tolerable. Rarely, however, an effect such as slowing of the sinus node can lead to severe bradycardia and syncope. If continued lithium therapy is a high priority, use of a pacemaker to provide cardiac stability could be considered.
- Through the dysregulation of calcium metabolism, lithium may cause hypercalcemia and hyperparathyroidism, which in

turn may lead to osteopenia, osteoporosis, bone resorption, and hypermagnesemia.

- Weight gain is another common adverse effect troublesome in long-term lithium treatment. Its mechanism is unknown. Patients should avoid caloric beverages, restrict food calories, and increase physical activity. Unlike the weight gain associated with medications such as olanzapine, lithium induced weight gain is dose-related. Therefore, reduction of the dose should be considered if the clinical situation allows it.
- Other occasional side effects of lithium are edema and a metallic taste in the mouth.

### ANTICONVULSANTS

Adverse effects that appear early in the course of valproate therapy are usually mild and transient, and tend to resolve in time. Gastrointestinal upset is probably the most common complaint in patients taking valproate and tends to be less of a problem with the enteric-coated divalproex sodium preparation. The administration of a histamine H2 antagonist such as famotidine (Pepcid) may alleviate persistent gastrointestinal problems (the metabolism of valproate is inhibited by cimetidine).

- Other common complaints include tremor, sedation, increased appetite and weight, and alopecia.
- Weight gain is even more of a problem when other drugs are administered that also promote weight gain, such as lithium, antipsychotics, and other anticonvulsants.
- Less common are ataxia, rashes, and hematological dysfunction, such as thrombocytopenia and platelet dysfunction.
- Platelet count usually recovers with a dosage decrease, but the occurrence of thrombocytopenia or leukopenia may necessitate the discontinuation of valproate.

Serum hepatic transaminase elevations are common, dose related, and usually self-limiting and benign. Fatal hepatotoxicity is extremely rare, is usually restricted to young children, and usually develops within the first six months of valproate therapy. Hepatic function should be monitored periodically during treatment as previously described.

Other serious problems include pancreatitis and teratogenesis. There is also a concern that polycystic ovary syndrome, possibly associated with weight gain, may be a risk for young women who take valproate. If at any point during administration the side effects of valproate become intolerable, the psychiatrist may need to discontinue it and try one of the other treatments described in this section as an alternative. If valproate is tolerated but not totally effective, the psychiatrist might use one of the other treatments as an adjunct.

Adverse reactions to carbamazepine (Table 3-12) are more likely if the dose of carbamazepine is built up rapidly:

- The most common effects in the first couple of weeks are drowsiness, dizziness, ataxia, diplopia, nausea, blurred vision, and fatigue.
- These tend to diminish in time or to respond to a temporary reduction in dose.
- Less common reactions include gastrointestinal upset, hyponatremia, and a variety of skin reactions, some of which are severe enough to require discontinuation of carbamazepine.
- Carbamazepine can be teratogenic and should be avoided during pregnancy.
- About 10% of patients experience transient leukopenia, but unless infection develops, carbamazepine may be continued.
- More serious hematopoietic reactions, including aplastic anemia and agranulocytosis, are rare.

Frequent blood monitoring, previously recommended, is generally considered unnecessary after the first few months of therapy. Instead, patients and their families should be instructed to contact the psychiatrist immediately if petechiae, pallor, weakness, fever, or infection occurs.

Carbamazepine has an antidiuretic hormone-like effect, which may help counteract the opposite effect (which produces polyuria) of lithium when the two drugs are used together. By itself, carbamazepine can cause hyponatremia. Gradual buildup of carbamazepine levels and smaller, more frequent dosing can help to minimize side effects, particularly in patients concomitantly taking other drugs, such as lithium.

Recently oxcarbazepine, the 10-keto analog of carba-mazepine, has become available as an alternative to carba-mazepine for the treatment of seizure disorders. Oxcarbazepine has less protein binding at 40%, and therefore less possibility for drug–drug interactions with highly protein bound drugs.

The only contraindication to lamotrigine use is hypersensi-tivity to the drug, though there is a box warning about derma-tologic events, particularly rashes.

- These rashes generally occur in approximately 10% of patients after two to eight weeks and are usually macular, papular, or erythematous in nature.
- Of those who develop a rash, one in 1,000 adults can proceed to a Stephens–Johnson type syndrome.
- Because it is impossible to distinguish which rashes will develop into this serious condition, it is advisable to discon-tinue treatment at any sign of drug-induced rash.

Otherwise the most frequently encountered side effects include dizziness, ataxia, somnolence, headache, blurred vision, nausea, vomiting, and diplopia. To reduce the risk of rash and other side effects lamotrigine must be started at a low dose and titrated slowly, especially if combined with valproate therapy.

### ANTIPSYCHOTICS

Although clozapine is free from most of the extrapyramidal side effects (EPS) associated with typical antipsychotics and may not cause tardive movement disorders, it does carry the risk of serious adverse reactions, including agranulocytosis, seizures, and cardiorespiratory complications. It should be used for bipolar patients only after other options have failed. Many experienced clinicians believe clozapine is superior to tradi-tional antipsychotics in the treatment of bipolar disorder, but definitive, controlled data are lacking.

Olanzapine has structural and pharmacologic similarities to clozapine but is generally less toxic. It shares with clozapine a low incidence of EPS and of hyperprolactinemia, as compared to typical agents.

- Adverse effects during the short-term use of olanza-pine include constipation, weight gain, akathisia, dry mouth, tremor, increased appetite, orthostatic hypotension, and tachycardia.

- The most common side effect is somnolence, which is why olanzapine is usually given in one q.h.s. dose.
- In clinical trials, there was a 0.9% incidence of seizures, and although there were confounding factors, olanzapine should be used cautiously in patients with known seizure disorders or lowered seizure thresholds.
- Because of alanine aminotransferase elevations in some patients, it is also advised to use olanzapine cautiously in patients with known or suspected hepatic impairment.

As mentioned earlier, maintenance therapy with atypical antipsychotics requires that careful attention must be paid to patient weight and blood lipid and glucose levels. This is partic-ularly true for clozapine and olanzapine but may also be true to a lesser degree for the other atypical agents.

- Weight gain on olanzapine may be as great as 5–7 kg though this plateaus in under a year. More modest weight gain occurs less frequently with quetiapine and risperi-done. Severe weight gain occurs in a minority of patients and, unfortunately, there are currently no means to predict whether a specific patient will experience significant weight gain. However, weight gain with atypical antipsychotics may be more clearly associated with a dramatic incrase in appetite, in food consumption, and in carbohydrate craving. It may be possible to evaluate patients for these features and be prepared to see alternative treatments if they occur.
- Atypical antipsychotics are also associated with hyperlipi-demia and with development of abnormalities in glycemic control (ranging from relative insulin resistence to dramatic and life-threatening new onset diabetes). Recommendations for monitoring metabolic parameters were discussed earlier.
- Some pharmacologic interventions which may reduce antipsychotic induced weight gain include addition of topi-ramate or of histamine-2 receptor blockers.

## DRUG INTERACTIONS

### LITHIUM
The narrow therapeutic index of lithium means that many pharmacokinetic and pharmacodynamic interactions are

potentially clinically significant, and several are associated with a high risk of serious toxicity (Table 3-13).

## ANTICONVULSANTS

The anticonvulsants have (predominantly pharmacokinetic) drug interactions due to the importance of hepatic metabolism for their clearance (Table 3-13).

- Valproate is metabolized by the hepatic cytochrome P450 2D6 system.
- Unlike carbamazepine, it does not induce its own metabolism or hepatic metabolism in general, but does appear to inhibit the degradation of other drugs metabolized in the liver.
- Valproate inhibits drug oxidation and may increase serum levels of concomitantly administered drugs that are oxidatively metabolized, such as phenobarbital, phenytoin, and tricyclic antidepressants.
- Coadministration of carbamazepine, or other microsomal enzyme-inducing drugs, will decrease plasma levels of valproate, and drugs that inhibit the P450 system, such as selective serotonin reuptake inhibitors, can increase them.
- The coadministration of other highly protein bound drugs, such as aspirin, can increase free valproate blood levels and precipitate toxic effects.
- Valproate increases the plasma concentrations of phenobarbital, lamotrigine, and carbamazepine, decreases those of phenytoin and ethosuximide, and may augment the sedative action of diazepam.
- Carbamazepine, phenobarbital, primidone, and phenytoin all decrease plasma levels of valproate, and salicylates can increase them.

Lamotrigine is metabolized predominately by glucuronic acid conjugation in the liver, with the conjugate and the remaining 10% of the unmetabolized drug excreted in the urine.

- Clearance is markedly increased with the administration of other drugs that induce hepatic enzymes—including phenytoin, carbamazepine, and phenobarbital.

■ **TABLE 3-13.** Drug Interactions with Lithium, Valproate, and Carbamazepine

---

## LITHIUM

| *Increase Lithium Levels* | *Decrease Lithium Levels* | *Increase Adverse Reactions* |
|---|---|---|
| Angiotensin-converting enzyme (ACE) inhibitors | Aminophylline (Aminophyllin and others) | Atracurium (Tracrium): prolonged neuromuscular blocking effects |
| Alprazolam (Xanax) | Caffeine | Carbamazepine (Tegretol and others): antithyroid effects |
| Amiloride (Midamor) | Carbonic anhydrase inhibitors | |
| Antipsychotic agents | Dyphylline (Lufyllin, Dilor) | Chlorpromazine (Thorazine and others): extrapyramidal symptoms, delirium, cerebellar function impairment |
| Ethacrynic acid (Edecrin) | Laxatives | |
| Fluoxetine (Prozac) | Osmotic diuretics | |
| Ibuprofen (Motrin and others) | Oxtriphylline (Choledyl) | Clozapine (Clozaril): neurotoxicity |
| Indapamide (Lozol) | Theobromine diuretic (Athenol and others) | Diltiazem (Cardizem): neurotoxicity |
| Indomethacin (Indocin) | Theophylline (Tedral and others) | Electroconvulsive therapy: confusion |
| Mefenamic acid (Ponstel) | | Fluoxetine (Prozac): lithium toxicity |
| Naproxen (Naprosyn) | | Fluvoxamine (Luvox): seizures |
| Nonsteroidal anti-inflammatory drugs (NSAIDs) | | Haloperidol (Haldol): neurotoxicity |
| Phenylbutazone (Butazolidin and others) | | Hydroxyzine (Atarax, Vistaril, and others): cardiovascular toxicity |
| Some antibiotics | | Iodine: antithyroid effects |
| Spironolactone (Aldactone and others) | | Methyldopa (Aldomet and others): hypertension, toxic symptoms at normal blood levels |
| Sulindac (Clinoril) | | |
| Thiazide diuretics | | Metronidazole (Flagyl and others): lithium toxicity |
| Triamterene (Dyrenium and others) | | Neuroleptics: extrapyramidal symptoms, somnambulism, neurotoxicity |
| Zomepirac (no longer available) | | |

■ **TABLE 3-13.** (Continued)

Pancuronium (Pavulon): prolonged neuromuscular blocking effects
Succinylcholine (Anectine and others): prolonged neuromuscular blocking effects
Verapamil (Calan and others): neurotoxicity

## VALPROATE

*Increase Clearance of Valproate*
Carbamazepine (Tegretol)
Mefloquine (Lariam)
Phenobarbital
Phenytoin
Rifampin (Rifadin and others)

*Increase Levels of Valproate*
Aspirin
Highly protein-bound drugs

*Valproate Increases Serum Levels Of*
Barbiturates
Diazepam (Valium and others)
Ethosuximide (Zarontin)
Phenobarbital
Phenytoin
Primidone
Tolbutamide (Orinase)
Tricyclic antidepressants
Zidovudine (Retrovir)

*Valproate Decreases Levels Of*
Carbamazepine
Lamotrigine (Lamictal)

*Valproate Increases CNS Depressant Effects Of*
Alcohol
Bupropion
Clozapine (Clozaril)
Haloperidol
Loxapine (Loxitane)
Maprotiline (Ludiomil)
Molindone
Monoamine oxidase inhibitors
Phenothiazines
Pimozide
Thioxanthenes
Tricyclic antidepressants

*Increased Risk of Hemorrhage With*
Aspirin
Anti-inflammatory analgesics
Sulfinpyrazone (Anturane)

## CARBAMAZEPINE

*Increase Levels of Carbamazepine*
Cimetidine (Tagamet)
Diltiazem
Erythromycin
Fluoxetine (Prozac)
Fluvoxamine (Luvox)
Isoniazid (Nydrazid and others)
Propoxyphene (Darvon and others)
Valproic acid
Verapamil

*Decrease Levels of Carbamazepine*
Phenobarbital
Primidone
Phenytoin (Dilantin and others)

*Carbamazepine Decreases Levels Of*
Antipsychotics
Benzodiazepines (except clonazepam)
Corticosteroids
Hormonal contraceptives
Thyroid hormone
Tricyclic antidepressants

*Other*
Lithium and carbamazepine:
may increase neurotoxicity

- Adding lamotrigine to carbamazepine can decrease steady-state concentrations of lamotrigine by approximately 40%.
- Adding lamotrigine to valproate, however, can decrease steady-state levels of valproate by approximately 25%, while the steady-state levels of lamotrigine increases approximately twofold. In this case, the starting dose of lamotrigine should be lowered, and the titration made slowly.

Concomitant administration of drugs that inhibit P450 will increase plasma levels of carbamazepine. Conversely, drugs that induce P450 enzymes—such as phenobarbital, phenytoin, or primidone—can decrease carbamazepine levels.

### ANTIPSYCHOTICS

Typical antipsychotics may interact with many other medications and the reader should consult the product prescribing information for further details. However, their use is declining in favor of the atypicals, the most widely used of which are olanzapine and risperidone. For effects of combining lamotrigine with other anticonvulsants, see Table 3-14.

- The metabolism of olanzapine and risperidone is induced by carbamazepine
- Levels of risperidone are increased by fluoxetine and paroxetine
- Levels of olanzapine are increased by fluvoxamine
- Neither olanzapine nor risperidone significantly interact with lithium
- Olanzapine does not interact with valproate; risperidone slightly increases valproate levels

■ **TABLE 3-14.** Effects of Combining Lamotrigine with Other Anticonvulsants

*Effects of Anticonvulsants on Lamotrigine Levels*
Carbamazepine decreases levels 40%
Oxcarbazepine decreases levels 30%
Phenobarbital decreases levels 40%
Phenytoin decreases levels 50%
Valproate increases levels 100%

## Pregnancy

All mood stabilizers are potentially teratogenic and the risks and benefits of treatment must be carefully assessed in the context of use during pregnancy and breastfeeding.

### LITHIUM

Exposure of a fetus to lithium in the first trimester has been associated with an increased risk of Ebstein's anomaly, a cardiac defect characterized by a malformation of the tricuspid valve. Data from a voluntary, retrospective source, the Danish Registry of Lithium Babies, provided an estimated relative risk for Ebstein's anomaly (compared to the general population) of 400. More recently, prospective cohort studies found risk ratios of up to 3 for all malformations and up to 7.7 for cardiac malformations. This corresponds to a risk of Ebstein's anomaly of less than 1 in 2000. This could be seen as a tolerable level of risk, particularly for a patient who has failed other mood stabilizer treatments and becomes rapidly very ill when she is not on lithium.

### ANTICONVULSANTS

Anticonvulsants as a class are clearly the most dangerous of the mood stabilizers to use during pregnancy. Fetal exposure in the first trimester to monotherapy treatment with anticonvulsants increases the risk of major congenital malformations 2–3 fold. When anticonvulsants are combined, the risk increases further. Valproate produces the greatest increase in risk of any individual anticonvulsant, being associated with major malformations at a rate several fold higher than other specific anticonvulsant, including carbamazepine. This excess risk associated with valproate is dose-related, becoming most evident at doses greater than 800–1000 mg/day. Among the newer anticonvulsants, lamotrigine has the largest prospective dataset. Rates of major anomalies were 2.9, 12.5 and 2.7% following 1st trimester exposure to lamotrigine alone, lamotrigine with valproate, and lamotrigine with other anticonvulsants, respectively. These data have been interpreted to suggest that lamotrigine has a risk no greater than other anticonvulsants and less than that of valproate. Similar to valproate, lamotrigine also produces greater rates of anomalies at higher doses. There is insufficient data at present to evaluate the risk of congenital anomalies following first trimester exposure to oxcarbazepine. The specific congenital abnormalities most closely linked to anticonvulsant exposure are neural tube defects, especially spina bifida. Use of folate supplementation may reduce this risk, but certainly does not eliminate it. As with congenital anomalies in general, neural tube defects occur with greatest frequency following valproate exposure (1–5%) relative to carbamazepine exposure (0.5–1%).

## ANTIPSYCHOTICS

There are less data available to guide risk/benefit assessment when considering using an atypical antipsychotic in pregnancy, but there is no evidence at present of any clear increase in the rate of fetal anomalies overall or evidence for the presence of any specific congenital syndrome associated with exposure. The typical antipsychotics have a much longer history of use in pregnancy and are also not associated with any specific syndrome. There is some evidence, however, that higher potency neuroleptics may be safer than lower potency agents.

## GENERAL PRINCIPLES

Because they are, of course, intimately interconnected, both the developing fetus and the mother must be considered in treating the pregnant women with bipolar disorder. Mood stabilizer discontinuation at any time is associated with an increased risk of relapse, which may lead to self-destructive or reckless behavior. In addition, we know from many preclinical studies that severe stress during pregnancy, in a range of species including primates, can produce long-standing abnormalities in the hypothalamic-pituitary-adrenal axis and increase the vulnerability to behaviors suggestive of depression and anxiety. Therefore, the ideal of minimizing exposure to medications during pregnancy may not always be the best option.

It is critical to carefully evaluate the potential risks and benefits of maintaining or discontinuing mood stabilizer treatment during pregnancy for each individual patient, in light of their need for specific agents and likelihood and speed of relapse off of medication. This must be done in a very open and comprehensive fashion, fully involving the patient and other important individuals, and emphasizing a thorough discussion of both the known risks and the limits of our knowledge. Ideally, options for pharmacologic intervention, if either elevation or depression intercedes, should be thoroughly discussed, in order to allow for the most efficient and informed intervention, should one be needed.

Another critical feature to consider is that the window of opportunity for medication discontinuation is very narrow with respect to the congenital abnormalities of concern with mood stabilizers. Cardiac development and neural tube closure occur relatively early, in the first trimester. Therefore, a patient presenting with one or two missed periods is likely already to be beyond the stage where medication discontinuation will be able to prevent increased risk. This argues for having a full discussion of risks with reproductive age women and a discussion about contraceptive methods being employed. Keep in mind, as well, that low potency oral contraceptives may be rendered ineffective by enzyme inducing medications such as carbamazepine.

Evidence from retrospective studies suggests that there is no protective effect of pregnancy on mood stability. In the immediate post-partum period, bipolar women are at markedly elevated risk of relapse. The most thorough study to date found a 90% relapse rate for unmedicated bipolar women in the first two months post-partum. Therefore, regardless of the decisions made during pregnancy, aggressive pharmacotherapy should be initiated in the immediate post-partum period.

## SUMMARY

Recent years have seen a remarkable increase in our understanding of bipolar disorder and the range of pharmacologic agents with which it can be treated. Lithium and valproate remain the core treatment options for bipolar disorder but are increasingly being supported by additional anticonvulsant and atypical antipsychotic agents. Although not definitively demonstrated yet, two relatively new medications, lamotrigine and quetiapine, hold significant promise as mood stabilizers with more robust antidepressant efficacy, helping to address an area of critical need. The increase in treatment options is simultaneously promising and challenging. It requires that clinicians learn to employ newer and older agents in the most rational manner, with decisions soundly based upon evidence of efficacy in clinical trials, as well as upon the individual clinical characteristics of each patient with whom we work. Carefully reviewing and documenting treatment response and tolerability is especially important in the unstable setting of bipolar illness, and can be aided by the use of clinical rating scales and daily prospective mood charting.

Even the best medication selection is of limited value by itself. A close, collaborative, and honest working alliance between the psychiatrist, the patient and family members, as well as a commitment to psychoeducation, is important for fostering trust, treatment adherence, and insight. Supportive psychotherapy techniques employed by a therapist knowledge- able about bipolar illness can also be extremely useful, helping patients to learn to properly differentiate normal emotions or reactions from affective symptoms, and promoting a healthy lifestyle with good sleep hygiene, reduction of stress, and avoid- ance of drugs and alcohol.

## ADDITIONAL READING

1. Keck, PE, Jr., Perlis RH, Otto MW, Carpenter D, Ross R, Docherty JP. The Expert Consensus Guideline Series: Treat- ment of Bipolar Disorder 2004. *Postgrad Med Special Report.* 2004(December): 1–120.
2. American Diabetes Association; American Psychiatric Associa- tion; American Association of Clinical Endocrinologists; North American Association for the Study of Obesity. Consensus development conference on antipsychotic drugs and obesity and diabetes. *J Clin Psychiatry.* 2004 Feb; 65(2):267–72.

# 4

# ANXIOLYTIC DRUGS

## INTRODUCTION

There has been an exponential increase in the number of medications demonstrated to be effective for the treatment of anxiety and anxiety disorders.

Barbiturates and meprobamate were some of the first agents shown to be effective in decreasing anxiety, but were addictive and often lethal in overdose. In the early 1960s, Klein demonstrated that the tricyclic antidepressant (TCA) imipramine was useful in the treatment of panic disorder. In the 1970s, studies showed that monoamine oxidase inhibitors (MAOIs) were also effective in the treatment of certain anxiety disorders, such as social anxiety and anxiety with coexisting depression.

The introduction of benzodiazepines in the early 1960s was a major advance; they were much safer than the barbiturates and meprobamate, had a rapid onset of action, and a broad spectrum of efficacy extending from situational anxiety to pathological anxiety disorders. Many different benzodiazepines, with different absorption times and half-lives, were developed and have been valuable not only for treating anxiety symptoms and anxiety disorders but for treating seizure disorders and alcohol withdrawal. Unfortunately, with wide-scale usage, problems with craving, dependence, and withdrawal with abrupt discontinuation were noted. The next major class

---

*Handbook of Psychiatric Drugs*   Jeffrey A. Lieberman and Allan Tasman
© 2006 John Wiley & Sons, Ltd

of agents approved was the azopyrones, of which buspirone is the most well known. This agent was effective in generalized anxiety disorder (GAD) but not for other anxiety disorders.

The selective serotonin reuptake inhibitors (SSRIs) as a class have demonstrated effficacy for most anxiety disorders. Although these agents have a delayed onset when contrasted with the benzodiazepines, they have a broader spectrum of action, no problems with dependence, and much less of a problem with withdrawal syndromes. Controlled trials have demonstrated the efficacy and safety of the selective serotonin-norepinephrine reuptake inhibitor (SNRI) medication venlafaxine in the treatment of anxiety disorders including social anxiety disorder, generalized anxiety disorder, posttraumatic stress disorder, panic disorder, and obsessive–compulsive disorder. Other classes of medications used in the treatment of anxiety disorders (either as primary treatments or as adjuvants) include anticonvulsants, beta-blockers, and atypical antipsychotics.

## A GENERAL APPROACH TO USING MEDICATION WITH ANXIOUS PATIENTS

Patients may present to physicians with many different concerns related to anxiety. Such patients commonly have the need for reassurance that their disorder is treatable, and that their physicians truly hear their concerns and will attempt to help them. Taking a complete history is essential not only for making an appropriate diagnostic formulation but for developing a therapeutic alliance. Medical evaluation, including laboratory testing, and assessment of current and past substance abuse or dependence, are particularly important in the evaluation of patients presenting with symptoms of anxiety. The differential diagnosis for such patients includes:

- Adjustment disorders secondary to life stressors
- Anxiety symptoms or anxiety disorders secondary to a medical condition
- Anxiety secondary to alcohol or substance abuse, dependence, or withdrawal
- Generalized anxiety disorder (GAD)
- Panic disorder (PD), with or without agoraphobia

- Social anxiety disorder (e.g., social phobia)
- Specific phobia
- Posttraumatic stress disorder (PTSD)
- Obsessive–compulsive disorder (OCD)

Sharing the diagnostic formulation with the patient is an important intervention that often facilitates the patient's commitment to the treatment plan. This is crucial since anxious patients may be reluctant to take medication. When they do take medications, they commonly ruminate about medication side effects. Patients with anxiety symptoms or anxiety disorders are likely to have somatic preoccupations and heightened somatic sensitivity. A collaborative approach where physicians and patients form a "team" to monitor both the potential benefits and risks of any medication intervention frequently enhances adherence. An important rule when initiating pharmacological treatment for patients with anxiety disorders is "to start low and go slow". Interestingly, although patients with anxiety disorders frequently require more gradual initial titration schedules, they often attain maintenance dosages of antidepressant medications that are greater than the doses used to treat major depressive disorder.

Along with medication interventions, psychoeducation about anxiety disorders is often a key part of treatment. In addition, psychotherapeutic interventions have been demonstrated to be effective in anxiety disorders, particularly cognitive-behavioral therapy, which may include cognitive restructuring, relaxation and breathing exercises, and graded exposure to anxiety-provoking stimuli.

## PHARMACOLOGY

### Antidepressants

It has long been known that antidepressants are also frequently effective treatments for anxiety disorders. The basic action of the majority of the antidepressants is to increase the availability of neurotransmitters in the synaptic cleft. The chemistry and pharmacokinetics of these agents are reviewed fully in Chapter 2.

The most widely used antidepressants with anxiolytic properties are the SSRIs. These agents have the broadest spectrum of activity which spans the entire spectrum of DSM-IV-TR anxiety disorders.

The mechanism of action of the TCAs again involves the inhibition of reuptake sites; their disadvantages include their side effect profile and their potential lethality in overdose. MAOIs can also be effective anxiolytics. The pharmacology of both groups of agents are reviewed in Chapter 2.

Other antidepressants with anxiolytic effects have different mechanisms of action. These include the inhibition of both serotonin and norepinephrine transporter sites (as seen with venlafaxine dosed above 150 mg/d, and with duloxetine and clomipramine); antagonism of the presynaptic alpha-2-adrenergic receptors (mirtazepine); and antagonism of postsynaptic serotonin type-2 receptors (nefazodone).

The relative differences in terms of major pharmacokinetic and pharmacodynamic properties are outlined in Table 4-1.

## Benzodiazepines

The benzodiazepines as a class work by increasing the relative efficiency of the gamma-aminobutyric acid (GABA) receptor when stimulated by GABA. They bind to a site located adjacent to the GABA receptor and cause an allosteric change to the receptor that facilitates the increased passage of the chloride ions intracellularly when GABA interacts with the receptor complex. This leads to a relative hyperpolarization of the neuronal membrane and inhibition of activity in the brain.

The benzodiazepines as a group have different affinities for GABA receptors; some agents bind to only one of the two types of GABA receptors. Both clonezapam and alprazolam work only on the central $GABA_A$ receptor, while diazepam binds to both $GABA_A$ and $GABA_B$ receptors. The pharmacokinetic properties of the benzodiazepines are outlined in Table 4-1. The half life of clonazepam is significantly longer than alprazolam (30–40 hours vs. 6–27 hours respectively); this is reflected in the longer time to steady-state plasma levels for clonazepam (up to 1 week). The relative pharmacodynamic

**■ TABLE 4-1.** Pharmacokinetic Properties of Psychotropic Medication Used for the Treatment of Anxiety Disorders

### SSRIs

| | Fluoxetine | Fluvoxamine | Paroxetine | Paroxetine CR | Sertraline | Escitalopram | Citalopram |
|---|---|---|---|---|---|---|---|
| $T_{max}$ h | 6–8 | 3–8 | 5.2 | 6–10 | 4.5–8.4 | 3–5 | 2–4 |
| Dose-proportional plasma level | No | No | No | No | Yes | Yes | Yes |
| $T_{1/2}$ (h) | 24–72 | 15.6 | 21 | 15–20 | 26 | 30 | 33 |
| Metabolite activity | Norfluoxetine (equal) | <10% | <2% | <1% | Desmethyl-sertraline 6–15% | None | <10% |
| Metabolite $T_{1/2}$ | 4–16d | – | – | – | 62–104 h | 50–60 h | – |
| Steady state plasma level | 4–5 wk | ~1 wk | 10 d | 10–14 d | ~1 wk | 10 d | ~1 wk |
| Usual daily dosage range | 10–80 mg | 100–300 mg | 10–60 mg | 12.5–75 mg | 50–200 mg | 10–20 mg | 10–60 mg |

### Other Antidepressants

| | Mirtazapine | Nefazodone | Venlafaxine | Venlafaxine XR |
|---|---|---|---|---|
| $T_{max}$ h | 2 | 1 | 2 | 5.5 |
| Dose-proportional plasma level | Yes | No | Yes | Yes |
| $T_{1/2}$ (h) | 37 (females), 26 (males) | 2–4 | 5 ± 2 | |

**■ TABLE 4-1.** (Continued)

**Other Antidepressants**

|  | Mirtazapine | Nefazodone | Venlafaxine | Venlafaxine XR |
|---|---|---|---|---|
| Metabolite activity | Negligible | Hydroxynefazodone | O-desmethyl-venlafaxine | C-desmethyl-venlafaxine |
| Metabolite $T_{1/2}$ (h) | — | 1.5–4 | 11 ± 2 | 11 ± 2 |
| Steady state plasma level | 5 d | 4–5 d | 3 d | 3 d |
| Usual oral dosage | 15–60 mg | 100–800 mg | 45–75 mg | 75–225 mg |

**Antianxiety**

|  | Buspirone | Alprazolam | Alprazolam XR | Clonazepam | Lorazepam |
|---|---|---|---|---|---|
| $T_{max}$ h | 0.6–1.5 | 1–2 | 5–11 | 1–4 | 1–1.5 |
| Dose-proportional plasma level | No | Yes | Yes | Yes | Yes |
| $T_{1/2}$ (h) | 2–3 | 6.3–26.9 | 6.3–26.9 | 30–40 | 12–15 |
| Metabolite activity | Unimportant | α-hydroxyl-alprazolam 50% | α-hydroxyl-alprazolam and 4-hydroxyl-alprazolam | No | Unimportant |
| Steady state plasma level | — | 3–4 d | 3–4 d | 1 wk | 4 d |
| Usual oral dosage | 15–90 mg | 1–10 mg | 1–10 mg | 1–6 mg | 1–6 mg |

### Antipsychotics

|  | Olanzapine | Quetiapine | Risperidone | Ziprasidone | Aripiprazole |
|---|---|---|---|---|---|
| $T_{max}$ h | 6 | 1.5 | 1 | 6–8 | 3–5 |
| Dose-proportional plasma level | Yes | Yes | Yes | Yes | Yes |
| $T_{1/2}$ (h) | 21–54 | 6 | 21–30 | 7 | 75–96 |
| Metabolite activity | No | No | 9-hydroxyrisperidone | Yes | Dehydro-aripiprazole |
| Steady state plasma level | 4–6 d | 2 d | 5–6 d |  | 14 d |
| Usual oral dosage | 5–10 mg | 300–400 mg b.i.d. | 2–8 mg | 20–80 mg b.i.d. | 10–30 mg |

### Anticonvulsants

|  | Gabapentin | Valproic acid | Pregabalin | Tiagabine | Topiramate |
|---|---|---|---|---|---|
| $T_{max}$ h |  | 4–5 | 1.5 | 0.75 | 4 |
| Dose-proportional plasma level | No | No | No | No | Yes |
| $T_{1/2}$ (h) | 5–7 | 9–16 | 6.3 | 7–9 | 21 |
| Metabolite activity | No | No | No | No | No |
| Steady state plasma level | 1 d | 7 d | 24–48 h | 2 d | 4 d |
| Usual oral dosage | 2,400 mg/d | 750–2,500 mg/d | 150–600 mg | 4–32 mg/d | 100–200 mg/d |

$T_{1/2}$, terminal half-life.
$T_{max}$, time of maximum plasma concentration.

and pharmacokinetic properties of the benzodiazepines are further outlined in comparison to the other medications in Table 4-2.

## Buspirone

Buspirone is believed to exert its anxiolytic effect by acting as a partial agonist at the 5-HT$_{1A}$ autoreceptor. Stimulation of the 5-HT$_{1A}$ autoreceptor causes decreased release of serotonin into the synaptic cleft. However, buspirone also exerts another effect through its active metabolite 1-phenyl-piperazine (1-PP), which acts on alpha-2-adrenergic receptors to increase the firing rate of the locus coeruleus. Some not yet *well-characterized* combination of these effects may be responsible for the anxiolytic effect of buspirone.

It usually takes approximately four weeks for the benefit of buspirone therapy to be detected in patients with GAD. A major advantage of buspirone is that it does not cross-react with benzodiazepines. The most common side effects associated with buspirone include dizziness, gastrointestinal distress, headache, numbness, and tingling. The pharmacokinetics and average daily dosage are described in Table 4-1. The most common pharmacokinetic and pharmacodynamic actions of buspirone are described in Table 4-2.

## Beta-Blocker Medications

Beta-adrenergic blockers competitively antagonize norepinephrine and epinephrine at the beta-adrenergic receptor (Table 4-2). It is thought that the majority of positive effects of beta-blockers are due to their peripheral (rather than central) actions. Beta-blockers can decrease many of the peripheral manifestations of anxiety such as tachycardia, diaphoresis, trembling, and blushing. The advent of more selective beta-blockers that only block the beta$_{-2}$-adrenergic receptor has been beneficial since blockade of beta$_{-1}$-adrenergic receptors can be associated with bronchospasm.

■ TABLE 4-2. A Summary of Pharmacologic Properties of Medications Commonly Used to Treat Anxiety

| | ONSET OF ACTION | TITRATION | ABUSE LIABILITY | NEED FOR DISCONTINUATION TITRATION | POTENTIAL FOR WITHDRAWAL SYNDROME | PROBABILITY OF LETHALITY IN OVERDOSE |
|---|---|---|---|---|---|---|
| Sertraline | Delayed (In 2 wk) | Yes | Very low | Yes, but not mandatory | Very low | Low |
| Paroxetine | Delayed (In 2 wk) | Yes | Very low | Yes | Moderate | Low |
| Fluvoxamine | Delayed (In 2 wk) | Yes | Very low | Yes, but not mandatory | Very low | Low |
| Fluoxetine | Delayed (In 2 wk) | Yes | Very low | No | Lowest | Low |
| Citalopram | Delayed (In 2 wk) | Yes | Very low | Yes, but not mandatory | Very low | Low |
| Escitalopram | Delayed (In 2 wk) | Sometimes | Very low | Yes, probably not mandatory | Very low | Low |
| Venlafaxine | Delayed (In 2 wk) | Yes | Very low | Yes | Moderate | Low |
| Duloxetine | Delayed (In 2 wk) | Yes | Very low | Yes | Moderate | Low |
| Mirtazepine | Delayed | Yes | Very low | Yes | Moderate | Low |
| Nefazodone | Delayed | Yes | Very low | Yes | Moderate | Low |
| Bupropion | Delayed | Yes | Very low | Yes | Low | Low |
| TCAS | Delayed (2 wk) | Yes | Very low | Yes | Moderate | Moderate–high |
| MAOIs | Delayed (2 wk) | Yes | Very low | Yes | Moderate | Moderate–high |

**■ TABLE 4-2.** (Continued)

| | ONSET OF ACTION | TITRATION | ABUSE LIABILITY | NEED FOR DISCONTINUATION TITRATION | POTENTIAL FOR WITHDRAWAL SYNDROME | PROBABILITY OF LETHALITY IN OVERDOSE |
|---|---|---|---|---|---|---|
| Buspirone | Delayed (2 wk) | Yes | Very low | Yes | Low–moderate | Low |
| Clonazapam | Rapid | Yes | Moderate | Yes | Moderate–high | Low |
| Alprazolam | Very rapid | Yes | Moderate | Yes | High | Low |
| Alprazolam XR | Rapid | Yes | Moderate | Yes | Moderate–high | Low |
| Lorazepam | Very rapid | Yes | Moderate | Yes | Moderate–high | Low |
| Diazepam | Rapid | Yes | Moderate | Yes | Moderate | Low |
| β-blockers | Rapid | Sometimes | Low | No (acute use) | No (acute use) | Low–medium |
| Gabapentin | Moderate (d) | Yes | Low | Yes | Low–moderate | Low |
| Risperidone | Rapid | Probably | Low | Yes | Low | Low |
| Olanzapine | Rapid | Probably | Low | Yes | Low | Low |

## Anticonvulsants

The precise mechanism of action of many mood stabilizers are not yet fully understood. Gabapentin, pregabalin, and viga-batrin increase brain GABA levels or neurotransmission at least in part by targeting the metabolic pathways of GABA. Tiagabine selectively increases synaptic GABA availability by blocking the reuptake of GABA via transporter inhibition. Evidence exists, to a greater or lesser extent, that all of these agents possess anxiolytic properties. See Tables 4-1 and 4-2 for a review of some of the more salient pharmacological proper-ties of these agents.

## Antipsychotics

Conventional or typical antipsychotics are rarely used as adju-vant medication for anxiety disorders due to problems with extrapyramidal side effects and the risk of developing tardive dyskinesia. The newer class of atypical antipsychotic medica-tions appear to have a decreased risk of these side effects and are beginning to be used as adjuvants in patients with treat-ment resistant anxiety disorders.

Although the different atypical antipsychotic medications have varying affinities for dopamine Type-$_2$ and serotonin Type-$_2$ receptors, this is the common mechanism of action of these agents. The atypical antipsychotic medications also differ dramatically in terms of their pharmacodynamic properties; a full review of these can be found in Chapter 1 and in Tables 4-1 and 4-2.

## INDICATIONS FOR USE

The efficacy of various psychotropic drugs for the treatment of anxiety disorders is summarized in Table 4-3.

## Antidepressants

### SSRIs

The SSRIs are considered the first-line treatment option for most of the anxiety disorders, including generalized anxiety disorder (GAD), social anxiety disorder (SAD), panic disorder

■ TABLE 4-3. The Efficacy of Psychotropic Medications for the Treatment of Anxiety Disorders

| | GENERALIZED ANXIETY DISORDER | SOCIAL ANXIETY DISORDER | PANIC DISORDER | POSTTRAUMATIC STRESS DISORDER | OBSESSIVE–COMPULSIVE DISORDER |
|---|---|---|---|---|---|
| Strong evidence | SSRIs<br>Venlafaxine<br><br>Trazodone<br>TCAs<br>Benzodiazepines<br>Buspirone | SSRIs<br>Bupropion-SR<br><br>MAOIs<br>Benzodiazepines | SSRIs<br>Venlafaxine<br><br><br>MAOIs<br>TCAs<br>Benzodiazepines | SSRIs<br>TCAs<br>MAOIs | SSRIs<br>Clomipramine |
| Some evidence | Nefazodone<br>Mirtazapine | Venlafaxine<br>Nefazodone<br><br><br>Gabapentin | Mirtazapine<br>Nefazodone<br>Clonazepam + sertraline<br><br>Buspirone adjunct to benzodiazepine<br>Valproic acid<br>Gabapentin<br>Tiagabine<br>Pagoclone | Venlafaxine<br>Lamotrigine<br>Valproate<br><br>Nefazodone<br>Mirtazapine<br>Clonidine | MAOIs<br>Olanzapine augmentation of SSRI<br><br>Risperidone augmentation of SSRI<br>Venlafaxine<br>Mirtazapine |
| Not effective | | TCAs<br>Buspirone<br>Pindolol augmentation of SSRI | Trazodone<br>Bupropion | | Trazodone<br>TCAs<br>Buspirone |
| No data | MAOIs<br>Bupropion | Trazodone<br>Mirtazapine | | Duloxetine<br>Bupropion | |

(PD), posttraumatic stress disorder (PTSD), and obsessive–compulsive disorder (OCD).

In GAD, paroxetine and sertraline have both shown efficacy in both adults and children, with symptom reduction and remission as measured by a variety of scales. Lower doses of sertraline are normally used for children with GAD and appear to be effective and well tolerated. Escitalopram has also been demonstrated to be effective in GAD.

SSRIs have emerged as first-line treatment for social anxiety disorder (SAD), also known as social phobia. Most of the efficacy data are derived from multicenter, double-blind trials of paroxetine, sertraline, and fluvoxamine. The use of sertraline for the longer-term treatment of social anxiety disorder has been investigated and shown efficacy in alleviating symptoms and prevention of relapse. Other SSRIs including fluoxetine, citalopram, and escitalopram also seem to be effective in the treatment of this disorder.

SSRIs are generally accepted as a first-line treatment for panic disorder (PD). The major advantage of these agents is their tolerability and thus longer-term acceptance by patients. At present there is evidence that fluoxetine, sertraline, paroxetine, fluvoxamine, and citalopram are effective in the acute treatment of panic disorder. Fluoxetine and sertraline have been shown to reduce panic attack frequency, global distress, and agoraphobic distress. Maintenance treatment with sertraline in one study was associated with continued improvement and protected patients from recurrence. Paroxetine has been reported to have a more rapid onset of action than other SSRIs in PD, and to show continued improvement over time. Citalopram and escitalopram are effective treatments of panic disorder, decreasing both panic attacks and phobic symptoms. Fluvoxamine has also shown efficacy for the treatment of panic disorder with or without agoraphobia.

SSRIs are effective for the treatment of PTSD, decreasing many of the core symptoms of this disorder. Fluoxetine was the first SSRI to be studied in randomized clinical trials, and showed significant improvement in both civilian and veteran populations. Two SSRIs have been approved by the FDA for the treatment of PTSD, sertraline and paroxetine. In one study, doses of sertraline of 50 and 200 mg/day gave sustained response; patients who responded during the acute phase not only maintained their response but continued to improve with six months of continuation treatment. Paroxetine in doses of 20 to 50 mg/day has been associated with treatment response across various types of trauma and in both men and women. Medication discontinuation has been associated with a significant risk of relapse and reemergence of the core symptoms of PTSD. This suggests that some patients will require sustained SSRI treatment, possibly for years, in order to protect them from exacerbation of their symptoms.

Large, well-designed, double-blind, placebo-controlled trials have demonstrated that the SSRIs fluoxetine, paroxetine, fluvoxamine, citalopram, and sertraline are effective acute treatments for OCD in both adults and children, as measured by a variety of severity scales. No significant differences have been noted between citalopram, paroxetine, and fluvoxamine, although citalopram may show efficacy in patients with treatment refractory OCD who were previously treated with another SSRI for at least six months. Sustained improvement has been shown with sertraline over a period of two years of treatment in both adults and children with OCD, and also appears to have a role in relapse prevention. Discontinuing SSRI treatment is associated with an exacerbation of symptoms and worsening in quality of life. These data suggest that SSRIs are a first-line pharmacotherapy for both acute and maintenance treatment of OCD in children and adults.

### SNRIs

In comparison to the SSRIs, there is less research demonstrating the efficacy of SNRI medications for treatment of anxiety disorders. In controlled trials, venlafaxine (particularly the extended release form) has been shown to be effective in the treatment of GAD, SAD, PTSD, PD, and OCD. For example, in one study of GAD, venlafaxine ER in doses as low as 37.5 mg/day and as high as 225 mg/day was found to be effective in decreasing symptoms of anxiety. Side effects appeared to be mild and tended to decrease in number and intensity over the course of the studies. Nausea, dry mouth, and somnolence were the most commonly repeated side effects. Venlafaxine

ER has also been shown to be effective in the short-term treatment of generalized social anxiety disorder. Its place relative to SSRIs in panic disorder is not yet clear; for instance, in a recent large study in panic disorder Venlafaxine ER treatment led to greater remission and fewer limited symptom panic attacks but not to a greater percentage of patients free of full-symptom panic attacks. Venlafaxine has been shown to produce improvement in PTSD symptom severity in some small studies.

Comparable studies on the use of duloxetine, a newly-released SNRI, in anxiety disorders have not yet been reported.


## TCAs

The tricyclic antidepressants have been demonstrated to have efficacy for many anxiety disorders, including SAD, PD, PTSD, and OCD, but not social anxiety disorder. However, the TCAs have significant side effects, may lead to more difficulty in dosage titration, and are potentially lethal in overdose. In addition, many anxiety disorders require long-term medication treatment. Since the significant side-effect burden of TCAs often leads to long-term non-compliance, and hence a greater chance of relapse, their use has diminished in recent years.

A variety of tricyclic antidepressants (TCAs) have been demonstrated to be effective treatments for GAD. Similarly, in panic disorder, numerous TCAs (particularly the serotonergic agents such as imipramine) have been shown to be effective for both acute and maintenance treatment of panic attacks. In PTSD, several TCAs (including amitriptyline and imipramine) have shown efficacy in decreasing signs and symptoms of that disorder. However, following the advent of SSRIs with their significant safety and tolerability advantages, PTSD studies with TCAs have not been pursued.

The TCA clomipramine is particularly effective in the treatment of OCD. Used in doses ranging from 100 to 250 mg/day, clomipramine has been shown to be as effective as the SSRIs and may, in some instances, be more effective in treating OCD symptoms. However, it is highly anticholinergic and sedating, unlike the SSRI medications, and more likely to lead to discontinuation.

## MAOIs

MAO inhibitor medications are efficacious in many anxiety disorders, but are not commonly used as first-line treatments because the need to follow a tyramine-free diet to avoid hypertensive crisis makes this class of drugs unappealing for most patients. For instance, first-generation MAOIs are effective in the treatment of social anxiety disorder, and may be more effective than the SSRI medications. These agents may be useful for severely ill patients with PD, particularly those with comorbid depressive disorder. A few small double-blind studies suggest that MAOIs are more effective than placebo in the treatment of PTSD. MAOIs have shown efficacy in some studies of OCD, but are not generally used as a primary treatment. Reversible MAO inhibitors such as moclobemide and brofaromine (neither is available in the US) are less likely to induce hypertensive crisis than first-generation MAOIs. They have also been studied in anxiety disorders including SAD and PD, and have demonstrated efficacy, though perhaps less than first-generation MAOIs.

### OTHER ANTIDEPRESSANT AGENTS

Anxiety disorders may respond to other classes of antidepressants, in general more variably than to the SSRIs.

***Bupropion*** Buproprion-SR has been found to be effective in the treatment of social anxiety disorder, and to be ineffective in PD, and also in an open-label study with PTSD.

***Mirtazapine*** Mirtazapine may be effective in the treatment of panic disorder and generalized anxiety disorder. Mirtazapine has also been studied in patients with chronic PTSD; results from small studies indicate it may also be efficacious as an adjuvant in the treatment of PTSD. In OCD, small studies with mirtazapine (as primary treatment or augmentation of SSRI medication) suggest possible benefit, even an acceleration of treatment response.

***Nefazodone*** The efficacy of nefazodone has been assessed in open-label studies in PTSD; results suggest that this agent may decrease the core symptoms of PTSD, improve sleep, and decrease symptoms of anger. It may be helpful for patients who are refractory to SSRI treatment.

*Trazodone*   Some older studies also suggest that trazodone is an effective treatment for GAD.

## Benzodiazepines

As a class, benzodiazepines are efficacious for the treatment of many anxiety disorders, including panic disorder, social anxiety disorder, generalized anxiety disorder, alcohol withdrawal, and situational anxiety. Although obsessive–compulsive disorder falls within the taxonomy of anxiety disorders, benzodiazepines do not seem to be particularly effective in treating these patients. The BZDs may be contraindicated in the ongoing treatment of PTSD; though open-label studies have suggested efficacy, a recent double-blind study found no benefit, and it is believed that BZDs may cause depression in such patients and potentially worsen the course of the disorder. There are concerns about dependency and stigma associated with the use of benzodiazepine medications.

Short acting benzodiazepines, longer acting benzodiazepines, and even the low potency benzodiazepines have all been demonstrated to be effective treatments for GAD. However, despite evidence that the anxiolytic effect does not tend to diminish over time and that the majority of patients do not abuse benzodiazepines, many physicians are reticent to initiate long-term BZD treatment for GAD.

The benzodiazepines clonazepam and alprazolam have been shown to be efficacious in treating social anxiety disorder. The potential for abuse and drug withdrawal is a particularly problematic issue in social anxiety disorder because of the high rate of comorbid substance abuse, and their use must be monitored carefully in such patients. Benzodiazepines may be best suited for patients with situational and performance anxiety on an as needed basis.

There is strong evidence that two high potency benzodiazepines, alprazolam and clonazepam, are effective in the treatment of PD. Alprazolam has been demonstrated in both short-term and long-term studies to be effective; however, there has been considerable concern about the risk of dependency and also the difficulties discontinuing alprazolam for a significant minority of patients. The immediate-release form of this agent has a relatively short half-life, requiring frequent dosing (up to four times a day). Recently an extended-release form of alprazolam has been introduced, with once-daily dosing.

Clonazepam at doses of 0.5–4.0 mg/day is effective and well tolerated in PD. Longer-term clonazepam treatment was associated in one study with continuing improvement and maintenance; the maintenance dosage was either constant with the initial response dose or decreased over time. There were no significant adverse effects associated with longer-term clonazepam treatment, though symptoms may recur upon discontinuation. Diazepam and lorazepam have also shown efficacy in treatment of PD.

## Buspirone

Buspirone has been shown to be particularly effective against the psychological symptoms of GAD such as worry, tension, irritability, and apprehension, but appears to be less effective in ameliorating somatic symptoms. The onset of action of this agent is at least two weeks; it may take three to four weeks before one sees a truly beneficial effect. Buspirone also requires divided doses to be effective.

Buspirone has been shown to be ineffective in the treatment of OCD, SAD, and PD, though it may have benefit as an adjunct to SSRIs in OCD.

## Beta-blocker Medications

Beta-blockers may be useful for individuals who have situational anxiety or performance anxiety. They generally have not been effective in treating anxiety disorders such as generalized social anxiety disorder, panic disorder, or obsessive–compulsive disorder.

These medicines are most useful for treatment of anxiety syndromes and disorders with somatic symptoms associated with increased adrenergic tone. Propranolol in doses of 10 to 40 mg/day has been used for performance anxiety, on an as-needed basis. Recent research on PTSD suggests a different role for the beta-blocker medications. It appears that traumatic memories may be reduced by medications that prevent presynaptic norepinephrine release (such as alpha-2-adrenergic agonists or opioids), or block postsynaptic norepinephrine receptors, blocking a cycle that is mediated by noradrenergic hyperactivity in the basolateral amygdala. There are two controlled studies of trauma victims presenting to emergency rooms suggesting that post-trauma treatment with propranolol can decrease subsequent PTSD symptoms.

## Anticonvulsants

Recent studies have suggested efficacy of the anticonvulsants gabapentin, pregabalin, vigabatrin (not available in the US), and tiagabine in anxiety disorders. However, further studies are warranted to determine if these medications should be used as monotherapy or as augmenting agents in individuals who are partially or non-responsive to conventional therapy.

Gabapentin at doses of 900–3,600 mg/day has been shown to be effective in the treatment of SAD.

Anticonvulsants such as tiagabine, valproic acid, and gabapentin maybe useful in PD with atypical or treatment resistant features.

In PTSD, open label studies of valproic acid, carbamezepine, and topiramate and a small double-blind study of lamotrigine have suggested benefit. Further studies are needed to determine whether anticonvulsant treatments will be beneficial in treatment of PTSD, either as a monotherapy or as an adjuvant with antidepressants.

## Antipsychotics

The development of the atypical antipsychotics has led to a reemergence of interest in their possible use either as a primary or adjuvant treatment for a variety of anxiety disorders. Small studies of risperidone and olanzapine augmentation in PTSD (also, quetiapine) in veterans showed some efficacy, however to date, the data are not overwhelmingly favorable for the use of atypical antipsychotic medication as either monotherapy or augmentation therapy for PTSD.

Currently, atypical antipsychotics are most commonly used in anxiety disorder treatment for augmentation of other treatments.

## Augmentation/Adjuvant Treatments

There is evidence that augmentation strategies can be effective in several anxiety disorders:

- Patients affected by OCD do not always respond to monotherapy with SSRIs or clomipramine; risperidone (initiated at 1 mg/day, titrating up to 3 mg/day over 2 weeks) and olanzapine (initiated at 2.5 mg/day and titrated up to 5 mg/day) may be useful in augmenting the clinical response in treatment refractory OCD.
- Buspirone may be used as an adjuvant to SSRI treatment for social anxiety disorder when patients exhibit only partial response to monotherapy.
- Buspirone may also be used adjunctively with a benzodiazepine in the treatment of PD.
- In PTSD, topiramate augmentation of SSRIs seems to be particularly useful in improving sleep, decreasing nightmares, and decreasing intrusive thoughts.
- Co-administration of sertraline (100mg/day) and clonazepam (0.5 mg/day) for PD has shown some efficacy.

## DRUG SELECTION, DOSE, AND INITIATION OF TREATMENT

The major initial choice in treatment of anxiety disorders is the class of medication. Initiation of treatment, dosage titration, and continuation of treatment as well as discontinuation depend on medication class (see Table 4-2). Even within a medication class (e.g., antidepressants), side effects may vary (see Table 4-4). Abuse liability, delayed onset of action, and probability of lethality in overdose may play a role in drug choice. Since anxiety disorders are often chronic, the long-term tolerability of medication is often another key factor in initial treatment choice. Generally single-agent treatment

■ TABLE 4-4. Common Reported Side Effects of Antidepressant Medications

| SSRI | SNRI | MIRTAZEPINE | NEFAZODONE | BUPROPION | MAOI | TCA |
|------|------|-------------|------------|-----------|------|-----|
| Nausea | SSRI side effects | Increased appetite | Sedation | Tremor | Dry mouth | Dry mouth |
| Decreased motivation | Dry mouth | Weight gain | Fatigue | Palpitations | Blurred vision | Blurred vision |
| Insomnia | Constipation | Sedation | Ataxia | Numbness | Insomnia | Constipation |
| Fatigue | Agitation | Fatigue | Dry mouth | Dizziness | Dizziness | Weight gain |
| Ejaculatory dysfunction | Diaphoresis | Agitation | Constipation | Spaciness | Orthostatic hypotension | Fatigue |
| Anorgasmia | Increased blood pressure | | Liver failure | Ataxia | Constipation | Sedation |
| Decreased libido | Weight gain | | | Seizures (in high doses) | Ejaculatory dysfunction | Orthostatic hypotension |
| Weight gain | | | | | Anorgasmia | Insomnia |
| | | | | | Anxiety | Hypersomnia |
| | | | | | Hypertensive crisis | Ejaculatory dysfunction |
| | | | | | | Initial jitteriness/anxiety |

is preferred initially, often using SSRI medication. BZD or other anxiolytics may be required during the weeks before SSRI medication takes effect, but can often be tapered at that time. Patients who are not fully treatment-responsive may require switches or augmentation of medication. Duration of treatment generally ranges from several months (for acute disorders) to a lifetime (for chronic disorders such as OCD). When medication is discontinued in anxiety disorders, there should be a gradual taper over many weeks to avoid rebound anxiety and to assess for the return of anxiety symptoms. The usual daily dose ranges for a variety of agents is shown in Table 4-1. In general, starting doses of 50% of the initial dose shown in this table are used for the first seven days of treatment.

Variations for some disorders include the following:

- Sertraline for treatment of GAD is usually initiated at 25 mg/day for the first week then titrated to 50 mg/day.
- Venlafaxine XR for the treatment of GAD and social anxiety disorder is usually initiated at 75 mg/day for the first week, increasing to 150 mg/day for the second week. Further titration to 225 mg/day may be needed.
- Gabapentin has shown efficacy at doses of up to 3,600 mg/day for social anxiety disorder.
- For social anxiety disorder, sertraline is usually initiated at 25 mg/day for the first week, then escalated to 50–150 mg/day.
- Doses of 20–30 mg/day of citalopram seem to be the most effective for the treatment of PD.
- Paroxetine is typically dosed at 20 to 50 mg/day for PTSD.
- Clinically effective doses for nefazodone in PTSD appears to be 400–600 mg/day.

## SIDE EFFECTS

The common side effects for antipsychotics, SSRIs, mood stabilizers, and benzodiazepines are given in Chapters 1–3 and 5 respectively.

Although a few individuals starting SSRI treatment may have some initial problems with restlessness and increased anxiety, data suggest that starting at lower doses such as

25 mg/day of sertraline or 10 mg/day of paroxetine may decrease the risk of antidepressant "jitteriness." This may be particularly helpful for patients with panic disorder, who may be acutely sensitive to the activating effects of SSRIs. Patients may experience the common side effects of SSRIs such as headaches, nausea, and diarrhea, however, most diminish with time and are well tolerated, particularly if the patients are informed of the possibility of these transient side effects.

The most common side effect of benzodiazepines is drowsiness, present in approximately 10% of patients. As a result, patients should be cautioned to be careful when driving or using machinery whilst on these agents. Residual daytime sedation often occurs the day after use of medication. Dizziness and ataxia can be experienced, which can lead to increased incidence of falls in the elderly.

Other rarer side effects can include:

- Maculopapular rashes and itchiness
- Anterograde amnesia (particularly with high-potency agents)
- Mild cognitive deficits

## DRUG INTERACTIONS

The common drug interactions for the antipsychotics, SSRIs, and mood stabilizers are given in Chapters 1–3 respectively. Combinations of drugs commonly used in treatment of anxiety disorders may lead to particular interactions. For instance, buspirone combined with other serotonergic drugs can lead to serotonin syndrome.

The most common interaction of the benzodiazepines occurs with other CNS depressants such as alcohol, barbiturates, tricyclic and tetracyclic drugs, opioids, antihistamines, and dopamine receptor antagonists. When BZDs are taken concurrently with other sedative agents such as alcohol, barbiturates or analgesics, marked drowsiness, disinhibition and respiratory depression can occur. Other interactions are shown in Table 4-5.

■ **TABLE 4-5.** Benzodiazepine Drug Interactions

| **Decreased Absorption** | **Increased Metabolism** |
|---|---|
| Antacids | Carbamazepine |
| Food | Rifampin |
| | Corticosteroids |
| **Increased CNS Effects** | Barbiturates |
| Antihistamines | |
| Narcotic analgesics | **Decreased Metabolism** |
| Tricyclic antidepressants | Cimetidine |
| Alcohol | Azole antifungals (ketoconazole, |
| Barbiturates | miconazole, itraconazole) |
| | Erythromycin |
| **Decreased CNS Effects** | Disulfiram |
| Methylxanthines (theophylline, | Oral contraceptives |
| aminophylline, caffeine) | Norfluoxetine* |
| | Fluvoxamine |
| | Nefazodone |
| | Isoniazid |

* Major metabolite of fluoxetine.
From Fogelman S and Greenblatt DJ (2000) Anxiolytics. In *Psychiatric Drugs*, Lieberman JA and Tasman A (eds.) WB Saunders, pp. 128–155. © 2000, with permission from Elsevier.

## CONTRAINDICATIONS AND SPECIAL PRECAUTIONS

Benzodiazepines may be teratogenic; their use in pregnancy is thus not advised. Their use in the third trimester may precipitate a withdrawal syndrome in neonates; in addition, they are secreted in breast milk in sufficient concentrations to cause drowsiness, bradycardia, and dyspnea in infants. The use of SSRIs in pregnancy and post-partum are detailed in Chapter 2.

The elderly and patients with hepatic disease are more likely to experience adverse effects and toxicity to benzodiazepines due to their reduced metabolism of these agents. Caution should also be used in prescribing these agents for patients with COPD and sleep apnea, a history of substance abuse, cognitive disorders, renal disease, CNS depression, porphyria, and myasthenia gravis.

Problems with tolerance, dependence or withdrawal are not usually experienced with short-term use of BZDs at moderate doses, although the short-acting agents may cause increased anxiety the day after taking a single dose. Some patients also

■ **TABLE 4-6.** Benzodiazepine Withdrawal Syndrome

| | | |
|---|---|---|
| Anxiety | Irritability | Perceptual disturbances |
| Insomnia | Tinnitus | Depression |
| Anorexia | Increased sensitivity to light and sounds | Autonomic overactivity |
| Vertigo | Headache | Seizures |
| Tremor | | |

From Fogelman S and Greenblatt DJ (2000) Anxiolytics. In Psychiatric Drugs, Lieberman JA and Tasman A (eds.) WB Saunders, pp. 128–155. © 2000, with permission from Elsevier.

experience a tolerance for the anxiolytic effects of benzodiazepines and require increasing doses to maintain remission of symptoms. Use of BZDs with longer half-lives (e.g., clonazepam, or extended-release lorazepam) may decrease these risks.

*Withdrawal syndrome*  The appearance of this syndrome depends on the length of time the patient has been taking a benzodiazepine, the dosage, the rate at which the drug is tapered, and the half-life of the compound. Abrupt discontinuation of agents with a short half-life is particularly associated with severe withdrawal symptoms, including depression, paranoia, delirium, and seizures. Some of these symptoms may occur in up to 50% of patients treated; however, severe symptoms only occur in patients taking high doses for long periods. Alprazolam seems to be particularly associated with immediate severe withdrawal and should be tapered gradually. The symptoms of benzodiazepine withdrawal syndrome are listed in Table 4-6.

## SUMMARY

Clinicians have a wide array of medications available for the treatment of anxiety symptoms and anxiety disorders. The breadth of treatment options available greatly facilitates our ability to help patients. We have safe and effective treatments for everything from the short-term treatment of anxiety reactions (such as an acute adjustment disorder with anxiety), to previously intractable and life-long anxiety disorders like

OCD. However, the most important therapeutic agent we possess is still sound clinical skills and judgement. Appropriate diagnosis and rapport are the foundations of any pharmacological intervention we make with our patients.

## ADDITIONAL READING

1. Nutt DJ, Ballenger JC. *Anxiety Disorders*. Blackwell Publishing, Malden, MA, 2002
2. Pitman RK, Delahanty DL. Conceptually driven pharmacologic approaches to acute trauma. *CNS Spectr.* 2005; 10:99–106
3. McDonough M, Kennedy N. Pharmacological Management of Obsessive-Compulsive Disorder: A Review for Clinicians. *Harvard Review of Psychiatry*, May 2002; 10:127–137
4. Blanco C, Antia SX, Liebowitz MR. Pharmacotherapy of social anxiety disorder. *Biological Psychiatry* 2002; 51:109–120
5. Bandelow B, Ruther E. Treatment-resistant panic disorder. *CNS Spectrums* 2004; 9:725–739

# 5

# SEDATIVE–HYPNOTIC AGENTS

## INTRODUCTION

Insomnia is a significant health care problem. The direct and indirect costs of insomnia are enormous for the entire industrialized world. Estimates of prevalence vary from 10 to 50% of the adult population, depending on the diagnostic, duration, and severity criteria used. An aging population, hectic work and personal lifestyles, and an increase in the frequency of nontraditional work hours (e.g., shift work) all may play a role.

Older adults, women and patients with underlying psychiatric disorders, such as schizophrenia, anxiety and mood disorders, are particularly prone to sleep difficulties. Treatment of the underlying psychiatric illness often improves sleep, obviating the need for hypnotics. However, some of the very medications used to control the condition could cause insomnia as well. For example, SSRIs may induce insomnia, while effectively treating an underlying depression.

## Diagnosis

Normal sleep consists of alternating episodes of rapid eye movement (REM) sleep and non-REM sleep. Non-REM sleep is further divided to 4 stages (stage 1, a brief transition between

---

*Handbook of Psychiatric Drugs*   Jeffrey A. Lieberman and Allan Tasman
© 2006 John Wiley & Sons, Ltd

wakefulness and sleep; stage 2, accounting for most of the time in non-REM sleep, features spindles and K-complexes on the EEG; stages 3 and 4, also called delta sleep, characterized by high amplitude, slow, delta waves on EEG, is thought to correspond to restorative sleep). Sleep latency, typically prolonged in insomnia, refers to the time it takes to fall asleep once in bed. In general terms, insomnia refers to the real or perceived inability to sleep, and presents as difficulty initiating and/or maintaining sleep.

Primary insomnia is diagnosed in the absence of any other sleep disorder (e.g., narcolepsy, obstructive sleep apnea), or those due to medical conditions or to medication or substance use. To formally make a diagnosis of primary insomnia, the DSM-IV-TR requires that the sleep disturbance last at least one month and that it causes significant interference in emotional, social, or occupational functioning. Polysomnography or actigraphy are not indicated for the routine evaluation of acute or chronic insomnia, but may be useful when sleep disorders such as obstructive sleep apnea or nocturnal myoclonus are suspected.

The more common secondary insomnia may be due to a variety of conditions such as hyperthyroidism, chronic pain, severe chronic obstructive pulmonary disease (COPD), restless legs syndrome, and/or medication (e.g., stimulants) or substance (e.g., cocaine, caffeine) use. Insomnia is also very common in patients with mood, anxiety, and psychotic disorders. Given the frequent co-occurrence, and that the direction of causality between insomnia and other conditions remains unclear, the 2005 NIH State of the Science Conference Statement concluded that secondary insomnia would be named more appropriately as "comorbid insomnia."

Although total sleep time could be increased in the elderly, the total amount of time spent in stages 3 and 4 sleep is reduced. The most common complaints of older patients, frequent awakening and the inability to sustain sleep throughout the night, results in less restorative sleep.

## Treatment Options

Treatment must be based on careful diagnostic assessment, including interview with a bed partner, review of sleep logs, and a diligent search for possible causes of secondary insomnia. Severe, chronic insomnia may only respond to medications, but non-pharmacological options should always be explored first. When indicated, hypnotic use is generally recommended for short-term use only. However, realistic alternative treatments to address the needs of patients suffering from chronic insomnia are not available. For now, basic sleep hygiene techniques, as summarized in Table 5-1, must be part of all treatments of insomnia.

## Non-prescription Agents

Over-the-counter (OTC) sleep aids most often contain the histamine ($H_1$) receptor antagonist diphenhydramine or some

■ **TABLE 5-1.** Sleep Hygiene Techniques

1. Do not go to bed when you are not tired.
2. Avoid napping during the day, even when you are tired. Especially avoid early-evening naps.
3. Wake up at the same time each day. Do not "catch up" on your sleep on the weekend.
4. Do not drink caffeinated beverages within 6 h of bedtime and minimize total daily use.
5. Avoid heavy meals too close to bedtime, but don't go to bed hungry, as this may disrupt sleep. A warm, noncaffeinated beverage and a small carbohydrate snack may be soothing and enhance drowsiness.
6. Regular exercise in the late afternoon may deepen sleep. Strenuous exercise too close to bedtime (i.e., 4–5 h) may interfere with sleep.
7. If you do not fall asleep within a half-hour or so, get up and read a book or watch television. When you stay in the bed and don't sleep for long periods of time, the bed becomes associated with not sleeping.
8. Minimize noise, light, and extremes in temperature during the sleep period.
9. Avoid the use of alcohol as a sleep-enhancer. Although it may promote sleep onset, early morning awakening is quite common and the sleep is generally nonrestorative in nature.
10. Use progressive muscle relaxation or deep-breathing techniques to enhance relaxation and minimize anxiety and stress.
11. Ensure that pain complaints have been appropriately evaluated and treated by your physician. Pain interferes with sleep.
12. Do not smoke cigarettes too close to bedtime or if you awaken in the night. Nicotine is a stimulant.

other sedating antihistamine such as doxylamine. They tend to have a prolonged duration of action leading to sedation and slowed reaction times the day after their use. Their side effects are substantial, including urinary retention, blurred vision, orthostatic hypotension, elevated liver enzymes etc. Tachyphylaxis often develops within several days to 1–2 weeks, limiting their utility to short-term insomnia problems. Unless pain is a significant complaint, the common practice of combining an analgesic such as aspirin or acetaminophen and an antihistamine (e.g., *Tylenol PM*) is no more effective than the use of an antihistamine alone.

Melatonin is a naturally occurring pineal gland peptide hormone available in OTC formulations. The FDA classifies it as a nutritive or dietary supplement. As dietary supplements are not reviewed by the FDA, the strength and purity of melatonin cannot be guaranteed. When taken orally, melatonin alters circadian rhythms, lowers core body temperature, and reduces daytime alertness. Melatonin may be particularly effective when the normal circadian cycle is disrupted (e.g., jet lag, shift work). Also unregulated, valerian may alleviate mild, short-term insomnia, but safety and efficacy have not been established.

## Prescription Medications

Benzodiazepines (BZDs) (triazolam, temazepam, estazolam, flurazepam, quazepam), and more recently, a series of non-BZD type hypnotics, or "Z-drugs" (zolpidem, zaleplon, es/zopiclone), have replaced most older hypnotics such as barbiturates, glutethimide, methaqualone, methyprylone, meprobamate, and tybamate. The replaced hypnotics were highly addicting and, due to their low therapeutic index, were also dangerous in overdose. In contrast, BZDs, and particularly the Z-drugs, are characterized by decreased abuse potential, fewer drug-drug interactions, broader therapeutic index, and lower risk in overdose. Daytime sedation and the risk for abuse and physiological dependence are the least likely complications of Z-drug use. BZDs and the Z-drugs are currently the most frequently prescribed hypnotics, but the off-label use (FDA-approved drug use for not FDA-approved indication) of sedating antidepressants (e.g., trazodone) as sleep aids, is common clinical practice. The melatonin agonist ramelteon, the most recently FDA-approved hypnotic in the US, is an agent with unique mechanism of action. The pyrazolopyrimidine indiplon, not yet available in the US, is also a non-BZD GABA/A modulator with promising side-effect profile. Other pharmacological options, limited to a few well-defined conditions with many caveats, include anticonvulsants (e.g., gabapentine, valproate, tiagabin) and antipsychotics (e.g., haloperidol, quetiapine).

## PHARMACOLOGY

### Benzodiazepines

All BZDs are central nervous system depressants via gamma-aminobutyric acid (GABA) agonism. Due to non-selective GABA binding, BZDs also possess anxiolytic, anticonvulsant, and myorelaxant properties. By modulating the effects of GABA, BZDs increase the frequency of chloride channel openings. In contrast, barbiturates and alcohol increase the duration of chloride channel opening. This seemingly minor distinction accounts for the greater safety of BZDs in overdose, with less likelihood of respiratory depression or coma. When alcohol is mixed with a BZD overdose, the synergism may result in fatal respiratory depression. Although effective hypnotics, BZDs significantly alter normal sleep architecture; daytime fatigue is probably related to reduced slow-wave, restorative sleep, while the memory problems reported by BZD users may be due to reduced REM sleep. REM suppression causes REM rebound upon BZD discontinuation, manifesting as vivid dreams and nightmares.

### Chloral Hydrate

Despite a rapid onset of action and relatively short elimination half-life, chloral hydrate, one of the oldest hypnotics, is rarely used as a hypnotic agent today, primarily due to its narrow therapeutic index. At dosages between 0.5 and 1.5 g, it is usually effective within 30 minutes. Chloral hydrate is metabolized in the liver and kidneys, and excreted renally. Chloral hydrate generally increases sleep stages 2 and 4, decreases stage 3 sleep, and has no effect on REM sleep.

## Zolpidem

The imidazopyridine zolpidem, just like all Z-drugs, is a BZD-like partial GABA-agonist with a non-BZD-like chemical structure. It is active at the $\omega$ receptor, which is a subunit of the $GABA_A$ receptor. BZDs activate all $\omega$ receptor subtypes. Zolpidem appears to bind preferentially to $\omega_1$ receptors. Although this selective binding is not absolute, it may explain the relative absence of myorelaxant, anxiolytic, and anticonvulsant effects at hypnotic dose, as well as the preservation of stages 3 and 4 sleep. Polysomnography indicates that zolpidem induces a sleep pattern similar to that of physiological sleep, and produces little disruption of sleep architecture following abrupt discontinuation. Zolpidem is rapidly absorbed through the gastrointestinal tract, reaching peak concentration from 30 minutes to 2 hours after administration. It is metabolized in the liver to several inactive metabolites and has an elimination half-life of approximately 2.5 hours.

## Zaleplon

Zaleplon, of the pyrazolopyrimidine class, also a non-BZD, binds preferentially to the $\omega_1$, $\omega_2$, and $\omega_3$ subunits of the GABA/A receptor. Peak serum concentration occurs within one hour of ingestion. Absolute bioavailability is only 30% as it undergoes extensive hepatic first-pass metabolism. Zaleplon is primarily metabolized by aldehyde oxidase and forms a number of inactive metabolites. Its elimination half-life is approximately one hour, making it an ideal hypnotic when insomnia is primarily due to the difficulty of falling asleep.

## Eszopiclone

The cyclopyrrolone eszopiclone, the stereoselective isomer of zopiclone, is the most recently (2004) marketed non-BZD "Z-drug" in the US. Due to rapid absorption and a half-life of six hours, it is indicated for both sleep initiation and sleep maintenance. Daytime residual somnolence and memory problems are much less likely with zopiclone, and probably with eszopiclone as well, compared to BZDs. Eszopiclone is the only hypnotic approved for long-term administration, based on a large, controlled treatment study that showed no tolerance to its hypnotic effect after six months of continuous use, followed by 12 months of open extension. Sleep architecture is only minimally altered; stage 2 and slow-wave sleep increase, REM remains unchanged. Polysomnography shows continued sleep improvement after drug discontinuation with no significant rebound insomnia.

## Ramelteon

This most recently FDA-approved hypnotic in the US, is a novel agent with high selectivity for the melatonin receptors MT1 and MT2. These receptors, located in the suprachiasmatic nucleus, have been implicated in the regulation of sleepiness and the sleep-wake cycle. Therefore, ramelteon may improve sleep through the endogenous sleep regulating system. With rapid absorption and a half-time of 90 minutes, ramelteon reduces sleep latency and increases total sleep time, with no residual sedation. Ramelteon does not appear to alter sleep architecture, and given the absence of significant side effects, even at significantly higher than recommended doses, its therapeutic margin seems wider compared to most hypnotics. If these reported properties, including efficacy, are confirmed in clinical practice, ramelteon should become the preferred first-line choice for the treatment of insomnia.

## DRUG SELECTION

In general, choosing the most appropriate hypnotic should be based on the type of sleep difficulty being experienced, the age of the patient, comorbid diagnoses, medical and psychiatric history, and concomitant medications used.

BZDs are effective for transient and situational insomnias, with reported improvement in sleep onset, number of awakenings at night, total sleep duration, and the quality of sleep. As doses, and consequently brain concentrations are increased, drowsiness and relaxation shift into decreased wakefulness and then sleep.

Although only five benzodiazepines are marketed as hypnotic agents in the US (Table 5-2), most BZDs induce sleep, provided an appropriate dose is chosen. There is no convincing evidence that marketed benzodiazepine hypnotics differ in terms of efficacy or safety when they are administered appropriately. They are similar in their effects on sleep architecture and differ only in onset and duration of action. Triazolam has a rapid onset and a short duration of action, making it appropriate for patients with sleep initiation difficulties, while flurazepam, with a longer onset of action and a much longer duration of action, is a better choice for patients with middle or terminal insomnia.

Shorter half-life BZDs cause less daytime sedation and residual cognitive effects, but may be associated with increased daytime, particularly morning, anxiety. Rebound insomnia upon abrupt discontinuation is common, especially after use for several consecutive nights, but can be avoided by gradual taper. The likelihood of rebound insomnia seems greater in patients who experience greater hypnotic efficacy. For at least some patients, this may reflect the development of physiologic dependence and a withdrawal phenomenon.

Longer half-life benzodiazepines, preferred for middle or terminal insomnia, often cause daytime sedation, decreased reaction time, and/or impaired coordination. Flurazepam and quazepam, with long half-life active metabolites, often accumulate with repeated administration, particularly in the elderly. Patients with significant daytime anxiety may benefit from the longer acting benzodiazepines, as the residual amount of medication left in the morning may still have anxiolytic benefits. BZDs are the preferred hypnotics for patients with insomnia and comorbid anxiety disorders.

BZD hypnotic use by the elderly, likely due to the greater prevalence of sleep disorders, is much more common than that in the general adult population. The elderly, as a group, have slower hepatic metabolism and less efficient renal excretion which is often more pronounced among men. In coordination, sedation and confusion can occur when longer-acting BZDs with active metabolites build up over time. Compared

**■ TABLE 5-2.** Hypnotic Agents

| GENERIC NAME | TRADE NAME | DOSE STRENGTHS (mg) | HALF-LIFE (h) | ONSET OF ACTION | COMMENTS |
|---|---|---|---|---|---|
| Chloral hydrate | Noctec | 500mg/5ml | 8–10 | Intermediate | Active metabolite trichloroethanol has CNS depressive effect |
| Triazolam | Halcion | 0.125, 0.25 | 1.5–5.5 | Intermediate | May cause anterograde amnesia |
| Temazepam | Restoril | 7.5, 15, 30 | 9–12 | Slow | No active metabolites |
| Estazolam | ProSom | 1, 2 | 10–24 | Intermediate | Active metabolite has weak sedating properties as well |
| Flurazepam | Dalmane | 15, 30 | 30–100 | Fast | Active metabolite desalkylflurazepam accumulates and causes additive sedation |
| Quazepam | Doral | 7.5, 15 | 25–40 | Intermediate | Same active metabolite as flurazepam |
| Eszopiclone | Lunesta | 1, 2, 3 | 6 | Fast | |
| Zaleplon | Sonata | 5, 10 | 1 | Fast | |
| Zolpidem | Ambien | 5, 10 | 1.4–4.5 | Fast | |
| Ramelteon | Rozerem | 8 | 1–2.6 | Slow | Unique MOA melatonin receptor subtype agonist |

to short-acting BZDs, much higher rates of falls and hip fractures have been observed in older patients taking long-acting BZDs; this risk increases in direct proportion to the daily dose. A generally safe clinical strategy when managing late-life insomnia is to halve the starting dose and titrate up slowly as tolerated following the longstanding advice "start low, go slow." Avoiding long-acting benzodiazepines appears prudent as well.

At present, conclusive evidence does not support clinically significant differences among the three available Z-drugs. Consequently choosing one over the others remains somewhat arbitrary. Quick onset of action and short elimination half-life may make zaleplon more appropriate for patients with difficulty in initiating sleep only. If maintaining sleep is also problematic, zaleplon's short half-life permits middle of the night or early morning administration without significant next-day sedation as well. Zolpidem and eszopiclone seem comparable in efficacy and in onset and duration of action. Both are likely to address difficulties in initiating and maintaining sleep. Compared to BZDs, residual daytime fatigue and somnolence are less pronounced during continuous use; rebound insomnia is rare upon discontinuation.

Ramelteon appears to least alter the intrinsic sleep architecture and therefore, if efficacy is established using active comparators, it may become the "ideal" hypnotic.

## Other Prescription Hypnotics

These agents have not been approved by the FDA for insomnia, but due to their sedating properties, they are considered useful alternative hypnotics in cases of treatment resistance, intolerable side effects, drug-drug interactions, certain comorbid conditions, current or past history of drug use etc.

At present, the most frequently used, non-FDA-approved hypnotic in the US is the triazolopyridine trazodone, marketed as an antidepressant. It is rarely used alone as an antidepressant because of its strong sedating qualities and the need for b.i.d. administration. Tolerance to its sedating effects develops only rarely with long-term use, making it an excellent option for those with chronic insomnia. In spite of a paucity of data in support of efficacy, trazodone is also the most popular choice to counter SSRI-induced insomnia. Hypnotic dosages vary markedly, from 25 to 300 mg, depending on individual susceptibility to its sedating effects. Trazodone increases slow wave sleep and total sleep time and does not appear to affect REM sleep. Its elimination half-life of between six and nine hours renders trazodone likely to cause daytime drowsiness. Using the lowest effective dosage and/or taking it in late evening rather than at bedtime may minimize this effect. Side effects also include hypotension and constipation, but priapism is exceedingly rare, occurring in less than one in 40,000 cases. Since anticholinergic side effects are not common, trazodone has some advantages over TCAs.

Small doses of sedating TCAs (e.g., amitriptyline, doxepin) are sometimes used as hypnotics. Patients with chronic pain may particularly benefit from this treatment strategy; TCAs are frequently used to potentiate the benefits of traditional pain medications. They are potent inhibitors of REM sleep, and their discontinuation is often associated with REM rebound. Anticholinergic and adrenergic side effects and toxicity in overdose must be weighed against potential benefits. Mirtazapine is a newer sedating antidepressant that targets both the noradrenergic and serotonergic systems. It may be a useful alternative to the tricyclic antidepressants as it is less anticholinergic and less toxic in overdose. Mirtazapine has strong antihistaminic activity that may cause significant weight gain with chronic use.

Hydroxyzine hydrochloride and hydroxyzine pamoate are sedating $H_1$ receptor antagonists that are used occasionally as hypnotic agents. Next-day sedation is a common problem with antihistamines as they have a relatively long elimination half-life. They are highly anticholinergic and may cause hypotension; they are not recommended as first-line agents for the treatment of insomnia.

Barbiturates, butabarbital, phenobarbital, and secobarbital, are still prescribed for insomnia, but mostly outside the US. Barbiturates are potentially lethal in overdose due to respiratory depression; they are highly addicting and their abrupt discontinuation may result in potentially fatal withdrawal reaction. Their use has generally been replaced by safer agents with much better side effect profiles.

Certain sedating anticonvulsants are reasonable third and fourth line sleep aids or add-on hypnotics for patients who do not respond or become tolerant to standard hypnotics. Bipolar patients suffering from significant insomnia may benefit from valproate, when BZD-type hypnotics are contraindicated, gabapentine or tiagabine might be good alternatives. Secondary insomnia due to restless legs syndrome may preferentially respond to dopaminergic drugs, such as pramipexole or levodopa. As a last resort, agitated elderly patients with dementia may preferentially respond to low dose sedating antipsychotics such as haloperidol or quetiapine. Although the new generation atypical antipsychotics are less likely to induce tardive dyskinesia, other complications like diabetes, obesity, and dyslipidemia suggest that the risks of using antipsychotics as hypnotics remain substantial.

## TREATMENT IMPLEMENTATION

It is always advisable to provide patients with information on good sleep hygiene practices (see Table 5-1). Although behavioral techniques such as stimulus control, progressive muscle relaxation, biofeedback, and sleep-restriction seem to complement pharmacotherapy, cognitive-behavioral therapy (CBT) alone may have better long-term outcome, compared to the combination of CBT and medications. In contrast, added CBT seems to facilitate the tapering of hypnotics.

When a hypnotic agent is prescribed, patients should be advised to take the medication on an empty stomach and with ample fluids (e.g., a full glass of water) to promote rapid onset of effect. For patients prone to nocturia, fluid intake should be limited during the hours before bedtime.

The clinician should always caution patients regarding possible side effects:

- potential impairments in memory, coordination, or driving skills
- unsteadiness if they are awakened after having taken a sleep aid
- tapering of medication before discontinuation; this will be required if medication is used for more than a few nights

- avoiding the use of alcohol when taking a hypnotic, as the effects are additive
- the propensity for medication abuse by patients with drug or alcohol problems

Universally accepted guidelines for dosing and duration of use for hypnotics are not established. Both dose and duration must be individualized with the goal of finding the lowest dose and the shortest duration. Short-term treatment (i.e., from one or two nights to one or two weeks) is reasonable for most patients.

Some patients with chronic insomnia may benefit from longer-term use, provided that there is careful monitoring by the prescribing physician. No criteria are presently available to identify this subpopulation. It seems reasonable to consider several short-term trials, with gradual tapering at the end of each period and a drug-free interval between each period, to establish the patient's need for and the appropriateness and value of continued therapy. Drug-free time intervals between initial treatment periods should range from one to three weeks, depending on the half-life of the agent and its active metabolites and the rapidity of the taper schedule. Re-evaluation of such a patient's continued need for hypnotic medication at 3- to 6-month intervals is also reasonable.

As the elderly are particularly susceptible to falls or confusion from hypnotic medication, use of the lowest available dosage strength is advisable. The elderly should also avoid the use of longer half-life agents or those with active metabolites with long half-lives because such medications tend to accumulate due to pharmacodynamic differences in drug metabolism in the elderly.

For individuals who prefer behavioral and nonpharmacological approaches to their insomnia, hypnotic use two or three times per week may be beneficial.

## ADVERSE EFFECTS

### Benzodiazepines

Shorter half-life hypnotics, particularly triazolam, appear to cause anterograde amnesia more commonly compared to longer half-life agents. Alarming reports in the lay press regarding a greatly increased risk of hallucination, confusion, and anterograde amnesia with triazolam use are not supported by all available data. All benzodiazepines can cause anterograde amnesia, particularly at higher dosages. Anterograde amnesia commonly occurs following benzodiazepine overdose. The prevalence of and the risk factors for anterograde amnesia with appropriate dosing of sedative–hypnotic agents remain to be determined. Other adverse effects are discussed in Chapter 4.

## Chloral Hydrate

Chloral hydrate has a narrow therapeutic index, causes gastric irritation, nausea, and vomiting, and, at high doses, may cause gastric necrosis. Overdose can be fatal due to respiratory depression. As with other sedative–hypnotics, dependence and tolerance may develop. Withdrawal symptoms upon discontinuation, particularly following prolonged use, include confusion, hallucinations, stomach pain, and severe anxiety. Long-term use may lead to induction of hepatic microsomal enzymes as well. Any concomitant medication with significant sedating properties should be used with extreme caution, as the effects are additive. When chloral hydrate is taken along with alcohol the effect can be supraadditive (as in a Mickey Finn or knockout drops).

## Zolpidem

The elimination half-life of zolpidem is prolonged in the elderly and in patients with impaired hepatic or renal function. Zolpidem is a partial CYP 3A4 substrate. Zolpidem overdose can cause respiratory depression or coma, especially when combined with other CNS depressants. The benzodiazepine antagonist flumazenil can reverse the effects of an overdose of zolpidem, reflecting its benzodiazepine-like mechanism of action.

Although zolpidem is classified as a schedule IV drug by the FDA, it appears to cause tolerance and withdrawal syndromes somewhat less frequently than benzodiazepine hypnotics do. Withdrawal symptoms occur more frequently if doses exceed

10 mg, the recommended maximum in the *Physician's Desk Reference* (PDR). Selectivity for $\omega_1$ receptors appears to be lost at higher-than-standard doses, cross tolerance with alcohol and benzodiazepines develops, and adverse effects are much more common. Anecdotal reports of hallucinations and confusion at standard hypnotic dosages should be evaluated across a spectrum of dosages and age groups.

## Zaleplon

Like zolpidem, this agent is classified as a schedule IV drug by the FDA. Higher than standard dosages have been associated with an abuse potential similar to that of triazolam. With dosages of 20 mg or less, abuse and dependence appear to be significantly less than that found with BZDs. Rebound insomnia has been reported, but it occurs less frequently than with short acting BZDs such as triazolam.

## Eszopiclone

Given its relatively recent FDA-approval, eszopiclone's side effect profile is yet to be assessed in clinical practice. Available information is largely based on its similarity to the mixed isomer zopiclone. Most similar to zolpidem, eszopiclone also seems to be associated with minimal daytime residual somnolence and significantly less rebound insomnia upon discontinuation compared to BZDs. In fact, elderly insomniacs treated with zopiclone demonstrated improved cognitive functioning in one study. Dosed between 1 and 3 mg, there is no evidence of tolerance or addiction after several weeks of continuous use. Since it lacks the respiratory depressant effects of BZDs, eszopiclone is not contraindicated in COPD.

## Ramelteon

A comprehensive and reliable assessment of the side-effect profile of ramelteon is also limited by limited clinical experience. Given its unique mechanism of action and seemingly least propensity to alter intrinsic sleep architecture, side effects should be minimal. The apparent absence of side effects at significantly higher than the recommended effective dose is particularly promising.

## DRUG INTERACTIONS AND SPECIAL PRECAUTIONS

Drug interactions with benzodiazepines are common. When mixed with other sedating compounds the effects are additive. Narcotic medications, alcohol, and antihistamines are examples where the additive sedation can lead to significant confusion. Alcohol ingestion slows hepatic metabolism and causes transiently higher concentrations of oxidatively metabolized benzodiazepines leading to further sedation. Antacids that slow gastric emptying may decrease the rate of absorption of a hypnotic agent from its primary site, the small intestine. This could alter both peak concentration and onset of effects.

Benzodiazepines all undergo some form of hepatic metabolism, although some agents are much more extensively metabolized than others. Medications that inhibit hepatic microsomal oxidative metabolism may cause clinically meaningful drug interactions when combined with benzodiazepines. All currently available triazolobenzodiazepines (e.g., alprazolam, estazolam, midazolam, triazolam) and diazepam are metabolized by hepatic microsomes and are complete or partial substrates of the CYP 3A4 isoform. Medications that are potent inhibitors of this system will cause higher peak concentrations of the triazolobenzodiazepine, particularly triazolam, which is highly hepatically metabolized. Nefazodone, ketaconazole, cimetidine, and macrolide antibiotics are examples of clinically relevant CYP 3A4 inhibitors which may cause a reduction in the clearance of these triazolobenzodiazepines and an increase in their blood and brain concentrations. This increase is greatest with higher hepatic clearance drugs such as triazolam or midazolam and somewhat less for drugs such as alprazolam or estazolam.

The CYP 1A2 isoform is also important in insomnia but from a different perspective. Methylxanthines (e.g., caffeine) and certain bronchodilators, such as theophylline, are significantly metabolized via CYP 1A2-mediated pathways. Inhibition of CYP 1A2 activity by the SSRI fluvoxamine or by certain fluroquinolone antibiotics (e.g., ciprofloxacin) in patients also ingesting caffeinated beverages or in those requiring theophylline may result in insomnia, agitation, or increased anxiety.

All benzodiazepine hypnotic agents are FDA Pregnancy Category X, meaning their use should be avoided during pregnancy, especially during the first trimester due to an increased risk of congenital malformations. A variety of congenital malformations, including cleft palate, delayed ossification of a number of bony structures, and an increased occurrence of rudimentary ribs have been reported. Chronic usage of benzodiazepines during pregnancy may lead to physiologic dependence and withdrawal symptoms in the neonate. The use of benzodiazepine hypnotics during the last weeks of pregnancy may result in neonatal central nervous system (CNS) depression, and their use during labor may lead to neonatal flaccidity. Nursing also poses significant hazards, as all benzodiazepines are distributed into breast milk to varying degrees. Since infants metabolize benzodiazepines more slowly than adults, accumulation may occur, leading to sedation and nursing difficulties in the infant. Pregnant women who have insomnia should be reminded of sleep hygiene techniques and given any hypnotic agent only with extreme caution. Diphenhydramine can be used with relative safety, but only for short periods of time since tachyphylaxis develops with prolonged use.

Benzodiazepines must be used in patients with obstructive sleep apnea only with extreme caution. Benzodiazepines may cause respiratory depression and can render patients less likely to mount an appropriate respiratory response to hypoxia. Zolpidem, zaleplon, or trazodone are less likely to cause problems for sleep apnea patients and may be preferable alternatives. Aggressive evaluation and treatment of sleep apnea [e.g., continuous positive airway pressure (CPAP)] is extremely important to ensure adequate restorative sleep.

Pharmacodynamic interactions between the Z-drugs and other medications are relatively rare, but cumulative sedative effects may occur in the presence of CNS depressants (ethanol, TCAs etc.). Compared to some BZDs that are almost entirely metabolized via CYP3A4, the Z-drugs are biotransformed by several CYP isoenzymes. Therefore, pharmacokinetic interactions with CYP3A4 inhibitors and inducers are less relevant. For instance, phamacokinetic interactions, involving the CYP-450 enzyme system, seem to be limited to increased plasma concentration of zopiclone when co-administered with carbamazepine or erythromycin and decreased plasma levels in the presence of rifampicin. Zaleplon has similarly uncomplicated drug interaction profile, as it is metabolized by aldehide oxidase. Since cimetidine inhibits aldehyde oxidase and CYP 3A4, and may increase zaleplon plasma concentrations by 85%, the initial starting dose of zaleplon should be halved in patients also taking cimetidine. Other potent inhibitors of the CYP 3A4 system such as ketoconazole and erythromycin also may increase zaleplon levels. In contrast, rifampin seems to increase zaleplon clearance.

## SUMMARY

Insomnia is common and disabling. Medical and psychiatric conditions are frequently associated with insomnia resulting in added impairment. Treatment of insomnia should be guided by careful assessment and needs to be individualized based on the specific needs of the patient. Effective non-pharmacological treatments are available and should always be considered first. Pharamcotherapeutic options have expanded dramatically over the past 30 years. Older agents have been gradually replaced by safer, more effective and better tolerated hypnotics. Benzodiazepines and a series of non-benzodiazepine hypnotics acting on specific subunits of the benzodiazepine GABA receptor are currently the most frequently prescribed hypnotics in the United States. A number of other medications with prominent sedating properties but FDA-approved indications other than insomnia are also available and safely complement the benzodiazepine-type compounds. Improved quality of sleep, fewer side effects, fewer drug-drug interactions, and the preservation of the intrinsic sleep cycle remain the primary goals of hypnotic-sedative drug development for the management of insomnia. At present, over 80% of those with insomnia problems are likely to respond to treatments.

### ADDITIONAL READING

1. Silber MH: Chronic insomnia. *N Engl J Med* 2005; 353:803–10
2. Roth T, Krystal A, Walsh J et al: Twelve months of nightly eszopiclone treatment in patients with chronic insomnia: assessment of long-term efficacy and safety. *Sleep* 2004; 27:A260

3. Buysee DJ, Reynolds CF, Kupfer DJ et al: Clinical diagnoses in 216 insomnia patients using the International Classification of Sleep Disorders (ICSD), DSM-IV and ICD-10 categories: a report from the APA/NIMH DSM-IV Field Trial. *Sleep* 1994; 17:630–37
4. Morin CM, Colecchi C, Stone J et al: Behavioral and pharmacological therapies for late-life insomnia: a randomized controlled trial. *JAMA* 1999; 281:991–99
5. National Institutes of Health State of the Science Conference Statement: Manifestations and Management of Chronic Insomnia in Adults. June 13–15, 2005. *Sleep* 2005; 28(9)

# 6

# PSYCHOSTIMULANTS

## INTRODUCTION

The psychostimulants methylphenidate, amphetamines, and atomoxetine reduce the core symptoms of childhood attention-deficit/hyperactivity disorder (ADHD) in approximately 70% of patients compared with 13% taking placebo. Short-term efficacy is more pronounced for behavioral rather than cognitive and learning abnormalities associated with ADHD. There is strong evidence for the efficacy of treatment in school age children but there is new evidence for efficacy in the treatment of ADHD in preschoolers, adolescents, and adults because of new large-scale randomized clinical trials for those age groups. Although psychostimulants are clearly effective in the short term up through 14 months, concern remains that long-term benefits over years have not yet been adequately assessed.

## PHARMACOLOGY

### Chemistry

Dextroamphetamine (DEX) and methylphenidate (MPH) are somewhat similar in chemical structure. Atomoxetine, the newest agent in this class, is structurally unrelated to the amphetamine derivatives.

---

*Handbook of Psychiatric Drugs*   Jeffrey A. Lieberman and Allan Tasman

- MPH (methyl-a-phenyl-2-piperidineacetate hydrochloride) has two asymmetric carbon atoms, resulting in four optical isomers: both *d*- and *l*-forms of the threo- and erythro- racemates. The threo- isomer is biologically more potent than the erythro- structure. The commercial manufacturing process produces the *d, l*-threo-MPH racemate exclusively.
- Amphetamine, (a-methylphenethylamine) is available in both *d*-amphetamine and *l*-amphetamine forms, as well as racemic mixtures. The DEX isomer appears to have more potent CNS effects and is preferentially used in most indications.
- Atomoxetine (*N*-Methyl-3-phenyl-3-(*o*-tolyloxyy)-propylaminehydrochloride) is also structurally unrelated to other agents in this class; it is formulated as the *R*(-) isomer.

## Mechanism of Action

The term psychostimulant refers to the ability of these compounds to increase CNS activity in some but not all brain regions. For example, while increasing the activity of striatum and connections between orbitofrontal and limbic regions, stimulants seem to have an inhibitory effect on the neocortex. Prominent central effects include activation of the medullary respiratory center and a lessening of central depression from barbiturates.

- The blockade of the dopamine transporter has been cited as the putative mechanism by which psychostimulants ameliorate ADHD symptoms.
- DAT blockade is now regarded as the putative mechanism for psychostimulants: radioligand binding studies have demonstrated the direct action of psychostimulants, particularly MPH, on striatal DAT.
- Preliminary data suggest a role for 5-HT mechanisms in some components of the ADHD syndrome, even though SSRIs have not been helpful in treatment.
- Postsynaptically, stimulants are direct agonists at the adrenergic receptor.
- They also block the action of a degradative enzyme, catechol-*o*-methyltransferase (COMT).

- DEX and MPH are thought to act differently inside the presynaptic neuron.
- Atomoxetine is a selective inhibitor of the presynaptic norepinephrine transporter, with no direct effect on serotonin or dopamine and minimal affinity for other norepinephrine receptors.
- Peripherally, sympathomimetics have potent agonist effects at alpha- and beta-adrenergic receptors: DEX stimulates cardiac muscle, raising systolic and diastolic blood pressure, with a reflex slowing of heart rate.
- Psychostimulants can also cause urinary bladder smooth muscle to contract at the sphincter and will increase uterine muscle tone and produce bronchodilatation.

## Pharmacokinetics

The pharmacokinetic characteristics of the stimulants are summarized in Table 6-1. Because MPH's short half-life prevents it from reaching steady state in the plasma, the standard tablet must be given several times a day to maintain behavioral improvement throughout the school day; a long-acting formulation is therefore preferred.

Atomoxetine has an elimination half-life of four hours in the efficient metabolizers (90% of the population). The pharmacodynamic reaction at the receptor, however, can last for 24 hours. The half-life of atomoxetine is greatly increased in 5–10% of patients who have a polymorphism at the cytochrome P450 2D6 isoenzyme that makes them poor metabolizers.

Pharmacokinetic studies show that the sustained-release preparations have properties different from those of the immediate-release (IR) tablets. The time course of peak plasma concentrations from the long-duration preparation depends greatly on the design of the capsule. OROS MPH has a slowly rising concentration over eight hours. The "beaded" long duration preparation, whether they involve MPH or amphetamine, provides an immediate peak and a second stimulant peak in plasma four hours later. A single daily dose of a sustained release formulation may therefore be equivalent to multiple doses of an IR preparation.

**■ TABLE 6-1.** Pharmacokinetics and Pharmacodynamics

| PARAMETER | DEXTROAMPHETAMINE | METHYLPHENIDATE | ADDERALL | STRATTERA |
|---|---|---|---|---|
| Metabolism | Hepatic to inactive metabolites | Extrahepatic to inactive metabolites | Hepatic to inactive or weakly active metabolites | Hepatic to low levels of active metabolite |
| Excretion | Renal, of metabolites; rate accelerated by acidification | Renal, of metabolites | Renal; rate accelerated by acidification | Renal (80%); largely as metabolites |
| $T_{max}$ | 2–4 h | 1–3 h | 2–4 h | 1–2 h |
| Half-life | 6–8 h | 2–4 h | 5–7 h | 5 h (21 h in poor metabolizers) |
| Effect onset | 30–60 min | 30–60 min | 30 min | – |
| Effect peak | 1–3 h | 1–3 h | 1–3 h | – |
| Effect duration | 3–5 h | 2–4 h | 3–5 h | – |

■ **TABLE 6-2.** Drugs for ADHD: Doses and Pharmacodynamics

| MEDICATION | TABLETS/DOSAGES | DOSE RANGE | ADMINISTRATION | PEAK EFFECT | DURATION OF ACTION |
|---|---|---|---|---|---|
| **Amphetamines** | | | | | |
| Dexedrine® | 5 mg | 10–40 mg/d | b.i.d. or t.i.d. | 1–3 h | 5 h |
| (generic) Adderall | 5, 7.5, 10, 12.5, 15, 20, 30 mg | 10–40 mg/d | b.i.d. or t.i.d. | 1–3 h | 5 h |
| (generic) Dextrostat® | 5, 10 mg | 10–40 mg/d | b.i.d. or t.i.d. | 1–3 h | 5 h |
| *Long-duration type* | | | | | |
| Dexedrine Spansule® | 5, 10, 15 mg spansule | 10–45 mg/d | once-daily | 1–4 h | 6–9 h |
| Adderall XR® | 10, 20, 30 mg capsules | 10–40 mg/d | once-daily | 1–4 h | 9 h |
| **Methylphenidates** | | | | | |
| Ritalin® | 5, 10, 20 mg | 10–60 mg/d | t.i.d. | 1–3 h | 2–4 h |
| Methylphenidate | 5, 10, 20 mg | 10–60 mg/d | t.i.d. | 1–3 h | 2–4 h |
| Methylin® | 5, 10, 20 mg | 10–60 mg/d | t.i.d. | 1–3 h | 2–4 h |
| Focalin® | 2.5, 5, 10 mg | 5–30 mg/d | b.i.d. | 1–4 h | 2–5 h |
| *Long-duration type* | | | | | |
| Ritalin-SR® | 20 mg | 20–60 mg/d | q.d. in am or b.i.d. | 3 h | 5 h |
| Metadate-ER® | 10, 20 mg | 20–60 mg/d | q.d. in am or b.i.d. | 3 h | 5 h |
| Medadate-CD® | 20 mg | 20–60 mg/d | q.d. in am | 5 h | 8 h |
| Concerta® | 18, 36, 54 mg | 18–54 mg/d | q.d. in am | 8 h | 12 h |
| Ritalin-LA® | 20, 30, 40 mg | 20–60 mg/d | q.d. in am | 5 h | 8 h |
| Atomoxetine | 10, 18, 25, 40, 60, 80, 100 mg | 0.5 mg/kg–100 mg | q.d. in am or b.i.d | – | – |
| Modafinil | 85 mg | 1.25–4.5 mg/kg | b.i.d. | 2 h | 8 h |

## Indications and Contraindications

The decision to use stimulant medication in the treatment of ADHD employs different criteria for each developmental stage. The criteria for use of stimulants in school-age children and adolescents are well described in DSM-IV. More difficulty arises when deciding whether to use these medications in preschool children, adult patients, patients with mental retardation, or children with ADHD and comorbid disorders.

### ADHD IN CHILDREN

The stimulants approved for the treatment of ADHD in children are summarized in Table 6-2.

New standards have been promulgated for the treatment of ADHD recommending multimodal therapy, and medication is one component of a therapeutic treatment plan. Other combinations, such as behavior modification plus medication, have been shown to be somewhat more effective than medication alone but medication plus cognitive–behavioral therapy is not more effective than medication alone.

Many stimulant treatment studies for school-age children with ADHD exclude children with full-scale IQs below 70, who are considered to have mental retardation (MR). This is unfortunate, for the signs of ADHD exist in children with IQs in the MR range. Treatment with a stimulant is effective in children with ADHD who have mild or moderate MR but they may be more vulnerable to adverse effects.

Stimulant treatment has also proved effective in children with fragile X syndrome and in children with pervasive developmental disorder, though the latter may be sensitive to stimulant side effects and may show increased irritability, motor activity, and stereotypies.

## DRUG SELECTION

- Different stimulant preparations share the same indications. Although MPH is regarded as the drug of choice for the treatment of ADHD, few controlled comparative studies have been conducted to determine which of these stimulants works best for which child.
- Pemoline, another medication for treatment of ADHD, has recently (December 2005) been withdrawn by the FDA.

Sustained-release preparations make it possible to give the psychostimulant once in the morning and avoid administration during the school day. There are three reasons for the implementation of longer-acting stimulant preparations:

• Children who take medications in school are subject to peer ridicule when they leave activities to go to the nurse.
• Some school officials refuse to allow school personnel involvement in the administration of medication.
• The time–action course of standard stimulant medications allows only a brief 1- to 3-hour window of effect, so some medicated children may experience trough periods of little or no drug action during important parts of the school day.

There are times when it is best to consider using nonstimulant medications in the treatment of ADHD. Possible criteria are:

• an unsatisfactory response to two different stimulants
• severe side effects
• psychosis is a definite contraindication for the use of stimulants.

Stimulant treatment has been associated with the appearance of reversible facial and shoulder tics for a minority of children. Even with these minor motor movements, most children can continue to be treated cautiously with low-to-moderate doses of stimulants, particularly MPH.

Other reasons for such a decision are listed in Table 6-3. Some alternative medications, including tricyclic antidepressants, bupropion, and clonidine, are listed in Table 6-4.

■ **TABLE 6-3.** Indications for Using Nonstimulant Drugs

Unsatisfactory response to adequate trials of both MPH and to DEX
Inability to tolerate stimulants
Comorbid condition(s) contraindicating stimulant treatment—e.g., psychosis
Medical contraindication—e.g., tachyarrhythmias
Risk of stimulant abuse by parent or other person in the home
When treatment of comorbid condition with a stimulant alone is not effective—e.g., tricyclic antidepressant for panic disorder and ADHD
Combination strategies for ADHD—e.g., tricyclic antidepressant plus MPH

■ **TABLE 6-4.** Non-stimulant Drugs in Attention-Deficit/Hyperactivity Disorder

| DRUG | USUAL DOSE RANGE | SCHEDULE | COMMENTS |
|---|---|---|---|
| Tricyclic antidepressants | 2–5 mg/kg; between-subject variability in levels at a constant mg/kg dose is common | b.i.d. or bedtime | Anticholinergic but generally well tolerated or mild and electrocardiogram precautions are mandatory<br>Consider therapeutic drug monitoring for side effects or lack of benefit. May be combined with stimulants |
| Clonidine | 0.1–0.4 mg | 2–6 times/day | Especially useful for comorbid tic disorders, sleep problems, and impulsive aggressivity<br>Monitor blood pressure<br>Tolerance and sedation are often problematical<br>May be combined with stimulants |
| Bupropion | 150–300 mg | b.i.d.–t.i.d. | Seizure history is a contraindication<br>May exacerbate tics |
| Atomoxetine | 100–300 mg | b.i.d. | Some weight loss may be experienced |
| Modafinil | 85–420 mg | b.i.d. | Some insomnia may result |

Atomoxetine fits into this treatment hierarchy as a second line medication, as shown by comparative trials against OROS-MPH. Trials with atomoxetine have lasted for up to one year in children and in adults. For those who respond, its efficacy during long-term use remains stable. Atomoxetine is indicated for the treatment of ADHD only as part of a comprehensive treatment program that includes psychological, educational, and social measures. In practice, atomoxetine can be used in children not on selective serotonin reuptake inhibitors after two stimulants have been tried; it may also be an option for families and physicians hesitant to use stimulant drugs because they are classified by the Drug Enforcement Administration as drugs of potential abuse.

## TREATMENT INITIATION AND DOSE TITRATION

- An effective treatment strategy for ADHD requires a plan for follow-up and monitoring.
- Techniques involve regular follow-up visits, the use of rating forms from parent and teacher, and the monitoring of academic progress in the school.
- Seeing the patient and a family member regularly is essential, often on a once-monthly basis when the medication prescription must be renewed.
- Once a child is diagnosed, the physician should have a systematic method for titration and adjustment of the dose.

Before the first pill is given, baseline data on height, weight, blood pressure, and heart rate should be collected as well as a complete blood count. The Conners Teacher Rating Scale and Conners Parent Rating Scale can also be collected. Standardized scoring methods for the teacher rating scale can be used to generate a hyperactivity factor score.

There is no universally agreed method for dosing and the dose may be selected according to the child's weight or by titrating the dose through the approved dose range until clinical response occurs or side effects limit further dose increases. Clinically, each child requires an individually constructed dose–response curve, taking into consideration the time–action effects of drug at each dose before making dosage adjustments.

Titration acclimatizes the child to the drug and determines his or her best dose:

* Children should be started with low doses to minimize adverse effects.
* Psychostimulant medication should be taken at or just after mealtime to lessen the anorectic effects; studies have shown that food may enhance drug absorption.
* MPH treatment can be initiated with a single 10 mg dose of long duration beaded methylphenidate at 8:00 am for 3 days; then a 15 mg dose at 8:00 am for the next 3 days; and finally 20 mg at 8:00 am for 3 days are given and maintained for at least 2 weeks.
* Preschoolers may start as low as 2.5 mg of MPH at 8:00 am but build to the same total 20 mg/day dose.
* DEX is usually started at 2.5 to 5 mg/day and gradually increased in 2.5- to 5-mg increments.
* The dosing instructions should be written down for the parent, with dates and times specified in detail.
* A photocopy of the instructions should be kept in the patient's chart.

The Conners Teacher Rating Scale is then repeated. Further dose adjustments up or down depend on the rating scale's scores, teachers' verbal reports, parents' comments, and adverse effects experienced by the child.

Stimulants with a shorter duration of action have been administered three times a day—before school, at lunch, and at home before homework. However, current practice is to start with a long-duration preparation, such as Concerta or Metadate-CD. This once-daily regimen avoids the noontime dosing in school. Eventually, a standard formulation may have to be combined with a sustained-release formulation at 8:00 am to ensure early- and late-morning coverage.

Plasma level measurements are not helpful for adjusting the dose of MPH because their inter- and intraindividual variability in plasma level concentrations are large and dose–response relationships vary from individual to individual. Adverse reactions to medications show the same variability and may appear unpredictably during different phases of the drug's absorption or metabolic phases.

Specific recommendations are made for atomoxetine:

- Atomoxetine is effective when given once daily but the total daily dose may be equally divided into two to reduce side effects, given in the morning and late afternoon or early evening.
- Treatment should be initiated at a dose of 0.5 mg/kg for children weighing under 70 kg; this should be increased over a period of three days to target doses of approximately 1.2 mg/kg.
- No therapeutic benefit has been shown at higher doses and the total daily dose should not exceed 1.4 mg/kg or 100 mg, whichever is the greater.
- For children weighing over 70 kg and adults, treatment should be initiated at a total daily dose of 40 mg and increased to 80 mg/day over three days; this may be increased after a further 2–4 weeks to a maximum of 100 mg if necessary.
- Atomoxetine should not be administered to patients with moderate or severe hepatic insufficiency.

## Treatment Evaluation

There is no agreement about:

- how many target symptoms must be reduced and by how much before a child crosses the threshold into "full clinical response";
- whether a full responder must improve in all settings (home, school, and the physician's office);
- whether response is best defined by clinician scored ratings or by parent and teacher ratings;
- whether impairment ratings, global ratings, or symptom scale scores produce the most valid and reliable indicator of response.

Each child's response to psychostimulants is different. Likewise, each family's needs are different.

- Maintenance plans should include schedules for the regular collection of information that constitutes the child's therapeutic drug monitoring.

- Dosing plans for the child's vacations, weekends, and after-school periods must be individualized.
- Many parents, concerned about long-term side effects, feel most comfortable with their child not taking medication each weekend and through the summer, despite the costs to family harmony. The benefits depend on the balance of behavioral problems and side effects in individual cases.
- Medication compliance should be monitored at each visit.
- Height and weight should be taken every six months, and the child's pediatrician can be requested yearly to perform a complete physical examination and blood work (complete blood count, liver function studies).
- The frequency of visits depends on the other therapies recommended. These may include once-monthly parental counseling, twice-monthly individual therapy, or weekly meetings for individual psychotherapy or behavioral modification management. A minimal frequency should be once-monthly, particularly in the nine states requiring multiple-copy prescription forms, which limit the amount of psychostimulant ordered to a 30-day supply.

A structured rating scale should be chosen that is easy to interpret, convenient to use, and available in both parent and teacher formats. These scales, however, should not be used as substitutes for an open discussion with the parent and teacher. They can be collected every four months or whenever the physician needs to make decisions about dosage adjustment, time of dosing, or even continuation of medication. Examples of these scales include:

- The 39-item Conners Teacher Rating Scale
- The ADHD Rating Scale filled out by the clinician

Current thinking indicates that a 25% drop from baseline in the mean of clinician-scored ADHD symptom ratings (with a lower total score indicating improvement) is defined as a positive clinical response. Once the maintenance dose of the stimulant is set, the rating scales for teachers and parents can be repeated at 4-month intervals.

## Maintenance Treatment

The predicted duration of treatment is an important step in the generation of a treatment plan for a child with ADHD. Although there is no clear-cut recommendation for the length of psychostimulant treatment, many parents have a reasonable expectation that it will not be open-ended.

• Treatment duration should be planned on an individual basis and planned in single school year units, starting with the present and projecting treatment to last through the present school year plus at least one additional month into the following academic year.
• Once the child has responded to an initial level of medication, maintenance doses can be set slightly lower. Treatment can be continued, if need be, and the next decision point can be set for the following fall.

A trial off-medication can be used to determine if treatment should be continued for another year. Medication can be discontinued during the school year, during some stable period. This should not be the beginning of the school year or during crucial placement examinations. Placebo tablets are no longer available from the companies producing MPH, so the psychostimulants are simply discontinued. Most children do not need to taper their dose of medication at discontinuation, unless they show signs of marked afternoon rebound.

## Treatment Resistance

Many apparent nonresponders to stimulants may simply have been treated with too low a dose or not treated with a second stimulant when the first one fails. Both MPH and DEX should be tried before moving to nonstimulant treatments for pediatric ADHD but specialist advice should be sought before venturing beyond a total dose of 60 mg/day of MPH and 40 mg/day of DEX.

• Approximately 25% of children with ADHD are not helped by the first psychostimulant given or experience side effects so bothersome that meaningful dose adjustments cannot be made.

- It is estimated that between 10 and 30% of children with ADHD do not improve with stimulants or improve but experience unmanageable side effects.

## Effects of Treatment on Symptoms

Stimulants ameliorate disruptive ADHD behaviors cross situationally (classroom, lunchroom, playground, and home when repeatedly administered throughout the day:

- In the classroom, stimulants decrease interrupting, fidgetiness, finger tapping, and increase on-task behavior.
- In the playground, stimulants reduce overt aggression, covert aggression, signs of conduct disorder, and increase attention during baseball.
- At home, stimulants improve parent–child interactions, on task behaviors and compliance; in social settings, stimulants ameliorate peer nomination rankings.

Although psychostimulants produce moderate to marked short term improvement in motor restlessness, on-task behavior compliance, and classroom academic performance, these effects have been demonstrated convincingly in studies where the medications are given under protocol conditions. For example academic improvement on tests of academic skills were maintained over 14 months of the MTA protocol. When examined over greater intervals, however, stimulant treatment plans in the community have generally failed to maintain academic improvement or to improve the social problem-solving deficits that accompany ADHD.

Unfortunately, there are only a handful of published treatment studies on preschoolers.

- MPH produces improvements in structured situations, but not in free play. Current labeling warns against using MPH in children below the age of six years. Even so, there was a 180% increase between 1991 and 1195 in MPH prescription written for preschoolers.
- MPH appears to have a linear dose–response effect on improvements in the mother–child interaction, perhaps related to increasing child compliance and decreased symptomatic intensity in the child.

## ADHD in Adults

The lifetime prevalence of ADHD in adults has been estimated to be at 4%, based on data from the National Comorbidity Study. Although it had been assumed that children
with ADHD outgrow their problems, prospective follow-up
studies have shown that ADHD signs and symptoms continue
into adult life for as many as 60% of children with ADHD.
However:

* Only a small percentage of adults impaired by residual
  ADHD symptoms actually meet the full DSM-IV childhood
  criteria for ADHD.
* Adults with concentration problems, impulsivity, poor anger
  control, job instability, and marital difficulties sometimes
  seek help for problems they believe to be the manifestation
  of ADHD in adult life.
* Parents may decide that they themselves are impaired by
  the same attentional and impulse control problems found
  during an evaluation of their ADHD children.

## Alternative Preparations to the Standard Stimulant Medications

The marketing of long-duration stimulant preparations was
preceded by a series of multisite, randomized, placebo-
controlled, parallel-design clinicial trials involving hundreds of
schoolage children. These trials were used for Phase 3 registration trials required for FDA approval. As a result, the stimulant
medication evidence base was expanded, and proved proof for
the safety and efficacy for mono-isomer MPH, racemic MPH,
and mixed salts of amphetamine.

 Second line medications have also been studied. The most
extensive controlled data exist for atomoxetine, involving over
a thousand patients in controlled trials, and 3,000 in safety
studies. Atomoxetine was the first agent in this class to receive
approval for ADHD in both children and adults; it improves
ratings of core ADHD symptoms in adults.

 The evidence for other medications is weaker. Fewer adults
studies have involved stimulants, as shown in Table 6-5.
Agents used for adult ADHD have included: MPH, 5 to 20 mg

■ **TABLE 6-5.** Experimental Medication Therapies for Adults with Attention-Deficit/Hyperactivity Disorder

| POSSIBLE MEDICATION TREATMENTS | SUGGESTED DOSE RANGE |
|---|---|
| Methylphenidate | 5 mg b.i.d.–20 mg t.i.d. |
| Amphetamine | 5 mg b.i.d.–20 mg b.i.d. |
| Mixed amphetamine salts | 5 mg b.i.d.–20 mg b.i.d. |
| Bupropion | 100 mg b.i.d.–100 mg t.i.d. |
| Selegiline | 5 mg b.i.d. only |

t.i.d.; DEX, 5 to 20 mg b.i.d.; methamphetamine, 5 to 25 mg once in the morning; bupropion, 100 mg b.i.d. to 100 mg t.i.d.; and selegiline, 5 mg b.i.d. only.

The evidence for the efficacy of these alternative stimulants for ADHD in adult patients is limited, so practitioners should be cautious in their use until more convincing proof is available. Of particular concern is the danger of using psychostimulants in adults with comorbid substance abuse disorder. It would be wise to use OROS MPH, because it cannot be broken down into a powder for internasal use, and because it has been shown in controlled studies to significantly reduce the symptoms of ADHD in adults. (See Tables 6-5 and 6-6.) Atomoxetine also has a low potential for abuse.

## Narcolepsy

Narcolepsy is a chronic neurological disorder that presents with excessive daytime sleepiness and various problems of rapid eye movement physiology, such as cataplexy (unexpected decreases in muscle tone), sleep paralysis, and hypnagogic hallucinations, which are intense dream-like imagery before falling asleep. The prevalence is estimated to be 90 in 100,000. Treatment can include a regular schedule of naps; counseling of family, school, and patient; and use of medications, including stimulants and rapid eye movement-suppressant drugs such as protriptyline. Treatment may begin with standard, short-acting stimulants, such as MPH, 5 mg b.i.d., and increasing the dose up to 30 mg b.i.d. if necessary. Modafinal is also indicated for the treatment of narcolepsy.

■ TABLE 6-6. Costs of Psychostimulants

| BRAND NAME GENERIC NAME | BRAND NAME MANUFACTURER | TABLET SIZE | DOSAGE RANGE | COST PER 100 TABLETS*: BRAND (GENERIC) ($) |
|---|---|---|---|---|
| Methylphenidate | Novartis Pharmaceutical, Summit, N.J. | 5 mg | 2.5–60 mg | 64 (25) |
| | | 10 mg | | 91 (35) |
| | | 20 mg | | 131 (69) |
| | | SR, 20 mg | | 198 (96) |
| | | LA, 10 mg | | 302 (NA) |
| | | LA, 20 mg | | 302 (NA) |
| | | LA, 30 mg | | 308 (NA) |
| | | LA, 40 mg | | 317 (NA) |
| Dexedrine (d-amphetamine) | SmithKline Beecham Pharmaceuticals, Philadelphia, PA | 5 mg (tablet) | 2.5–40 mg | 54 (28) |
| | | 5 mg (spansule) | | 130 (79) |
| | | 10 mg (spansule) | | 162 (98) |
| | | 15 mg (spansule) | | 207 (125) |
| Adderall | Shire Richwood Inc., Florence, KY | 5 mg | 5–40 mg | 227 (61) |
| | | 7.5 mg | | 227 (143) |

**TABLE 6-6.** (Continued)

| BRAND NAME GENERIC NAME | BRAND NAME MANUFACTURER | TABLET SIZE | DOSAGE RANGE | COST PER 100 TABLETS*: BRAND (GENERIC) ($) |
|---|---|---|---|---|
| | | 10 mg | | 227 (61) |
| | | 12.5 mg | | 227 (143) |
| | | 15 mg | | 227 (143) |
| | | 20 mg | | 227 (61) |
| | | 30 mg | | 227 (61) |
| | | XR, 5, 10, 15, 20, 25, 30 mg | | 373 (NA) |
| Strattera (atomoxetine) | Eli Lilly & Company, Indianapolis, IN | 10 mg | [0.5 mg/kg]–100 mg | 375 (NA) |
| | | 18 mg | | 375 (NA) |
| | | 25 mg | | 375 (NA) |
| | | 40 mg | | 385 (NA) |
| | | 60 mg | | 385 (NA) |

*SR*, Sustained release; *LA*, Long Acting; *XR*, extended release; *NA*, not available in this form.

* Prices are estimates based on 2006 Cardinal Health wholesale price guide provided by Pharmacy Department of New York State Psychiatric Institute, New York, NY, rounded to the nearest whole dollar.

## Other Indications

Psychostimulants have been used to treat depression, as a provocative test in schizophrenia, and to treat the cognitive–affective dysfunction found in patients with acquired immun-odeficiency syndrome-related complex. Anecdotal reports, open studies, and small controlled studies suggest that stim-ulants may help patients with depression and mania; in geri-atric patients who are withdrawn and apathetic; medically ill patients who are depressed; and in patients with patholog-ical fatigue or neurasthenia. Open studies using 20 mg/day of MPH as an adjuvant to tricyclic antidepressants in refrac-tory depression showed improvement, probably because of an elevation in plasma level of tricyclic antidepressants. However, controlled studies have not been done to show that combina-tion tricyclic antidepressant–stimulant regimens do better than tricyclic antidepressants alone.

## Costs

The costs of the principle treatments for ADHD are summa-rized in Table 6-6.

## ADVERSE EFFECTS

Stimulant side effects are dose-dependent and range from mild to moderate in most children (Table 6-7). Management

■ TABLE 6-7. Stimulant Side Effects and Their Management

| SIDE EFFECT | MANAGEMENT |
| --- | --- |
| For all side effects | Unless severe, allow 7–10 days for tolerance to develop. |
| | Evaluate dose–response relationships. |
| | Evaluate time–action effects and then adjust dosing intervals or switch to sustained-release preparation. |
| | Evaluate for concurrent conditions, including comorbidities and environmental stressors. |
| | Consider switching stimulant drug. |
| Anorexia or dyspepsia | Administer before, during, or after meals. |
| | With atomoxetine, consider drug-induced jaundice. |

■ **TABLE 6-7.** (Continued)

| SIDE EFFECT | MANAGEMENT |
|---|---|
| Weight loss | Give drug after breakfast and after lunch. |
| | Implement calorie enhancement strategies. |
| | Give brief drug holidays. |
| Slowed growth | Apply weight loss remedies, such as late-night snacks. |
| | Give weekend and vacation (longer) drug holidays. |
| | Consider another stimulant or nonstimulant drug. |
| Dizziness | Monitor blood pressure and pulse. |
| | Encourage adequate hydration. |
| | If associated with only $T_{max}$, change to sustained-release preparation. |
| Insomnia or nightmares | Administer earlier in day. |
| | Omit or reduce last dose. |
| | If giving sustained preparation, switch to IR preparation. |
| | Consider adjunctive antihistamine or clonidine. |
| Dysphoric mood or emotional constriction | Reduce dose or switch to long-acting preparation. |
| | Switch stimulants. |
| | Consider treatment of comorbid condition requiring alternative or adjunctive therapies. |
| Rebound | Switch to sustained-release preparation. |
| | Combine long- and short-acting preparations. |
| Tics | Firmly establish correlation between tics and pharmacotherapy by examining dose–response relationship, including no-medication condition. |
| | If tics are mild and abate after 7–10 days with medications, reconsider risks and benefits of continued stimulant treatment and renew informed consent. |
| | Switch stimulants. |
| | Consider nonstimulant treatment (e.g., clonidine or tricyclic antidepressant). |
| | If tic disorder and ADHD are severe, consider combining stimulant with a high-potency neuroleptic. |
| Psychosis | Discontinue stimulant treatment. |
| | Assess for comorbid thought disorder. |
| | Consider alternative treatments. |

generally involves a temporary reduction of dose or a change in time of dosing. MPH has an excellent safety record, probably because the duration of action of standard formulations is so brief.

Appetite suppression can appear when children with ADHD begin stimulant treatment. For this reason, dosing should optimally occur after breakfast and lunch. Even though the daytime appetite is reduced, hunger rebounds in the evening.

- The effects on appetite often weaken within the first six weeks of treatment and are reversed when treatment is discontinued.
- DEX, whose half-life is two to three times that of MPH, produces more sustained effects than MPH on weight velocity.
- MPH-treated children with ADHD followed up for two to four years show dose-related decreases in weight velocity, with some tolerance to the suppressive effect developing in the second year.
- About 20% of children treated with 1.2 mg/kg/day of atomoxetine lose 3.5% of their body weight; long-term follow-up over 18 months reported slight decreases in height and weight percentiles.

Height and weight should be measured at 6-month intervals during stimulant treatment and recorded on age-adjusted growth forms to determine the presence of a drug-related reduction in height or weight velocity. If such a decrement is discovered during maintenance therapy with psychostimulants, a reduction in dosage or change to another class of medication can be carried out.

The safety of stimulants in preschoolers is now under study. Although no multiple-sample pharmacokinetic studies have been done in preschool children to determine if younger children, with their larger liver-to-body size ratio, might require different doses for maximum efficacy and safety, one multisite controlled trial revealed that the optimal total daily dose of MPH ranged around 15 mg of the immediate release preparation. Therefore, it is wise to start preschool children with ADHD on low doses of the IR preparation. The study also

■ **TABLE 6-8.** Side Effects Associated with Atomoxetine

abdominal pain
decreased appetite
vomiting
nausea
somnolence
fatigue
sexual dysfunction (erectile dysfunction, impotence, abnormal
  orgasm)
loss of body weight
slight decreases in height and weight percentiles over 18 months
increased risk of mydriasis
allergic reactions, including angioneurotic edema
very rare cases of severe liver injury.

showed higher rates of adverse events in the younger group, even on lower doses of MPH.

The incidence of atomoxetine side effects in school age children appears to be low but comparative trials with other treatments for ADHD are lacking (Table 6-8). Atomoxetine has recently been found to cause rare cases of jaundice. Treatment with atomoxetine should be discontinued if hepatotoxicity is suspected.

## DRUG INTERACTIONS

Interactions between psychostimulants and other medications may be pharmacokinetic or pharmacodynamic and are potentially serious (Table 6-9). In particular, the addition of a

■ **TABLE 6-9.** Drug Interactions

| MEDICATION | STIMULANT | EFFECT |
|---|---|---|
| Guanethidine | MPH | Decreased hypotensive effect of guanethidine |
| Coumarin | MPH | Decreased metabolism of coumarin |
| Antiepileptic medications (phenobarbital, diphenylhydantoin, primidone) | MPH | Decreased metabolism of antiepileptic agents |

| | | |
|---|---|---|
| Phenylbutazone | MPH | Decreased metabolism of phenylbutazone |
| Tricyclic antidepressants | MPH | Decreased metabolism of antidepressant |
| Ammonium chloride | DEX | Increased elimination of DEX |
| Sodium phosphate | DEX | Increased elimination of DEX |
| Acetazolamide | DEX | Delayed elimination of DEX |
| Thiazide diuretics | DEX | Delayed elimination of DEX |
| Sympathomimetics | MPH, DEX | Increased sympathomimetic effects |
| Sympatholytic antihypertensives (beta blockers, others) | MPH, DEX | Decreased antihypertensive effect of antihypertensives |
| Albuterol | atomoxetine | Potentiates increased heart rate and blood pressure |

From Waslick B and Greenhill LL (2000) Psychostimulants. In *Psychiatric Drugs*, Lieberman JA and Tasman A (eds.) WB Saunders, pp. 128–155. © 2000, with permission from Elsevier.

psychostimulant to a monoamine oxidase inhibitor antidepressant regimen is a potentially lethal combination that can elevate blood pressure to dangerous levels. Other medications have been combined successfully with MPH, such as clonazepam to reduce tics and clonidine to reduce sleep disturbances.

## SUMMARY

Psychostimulant medications are a mainstay in the treatment of ADHD. This popularity has resulted from their proven efficacy during short-term controlled studies, as shown by lower ADHD symptom scores given by teachers and parents. In fact, the majority of children with ADHD respond to either MPH or DEX, so nonresponders are infrequent. Yet, the response of ADHD children to MPH and other psychostimulants for more than two years is not yet known. Optimal treatment involves the planning for a multimodal treatment program that combines educational and psychosocial interventions with medication therapy.

However, treatment plans that center on psychostimulant medication have flourished for a number of reasons.

The effects of psychostimulants are rapid, dramatic, and normalizing. The risk of long-term side effects remains low, and no substantial impairments have emerged to lessen the remarkable therapeutic benefit–risk ratio of these medications. More expensive and demanding treatments, including behavior modification and cognitive–behavioral therapies, have, at best, only equaled the treatment with psychostimulants. In the MTA study, the combination of behavioral and medication therapies was only slightly more effective than the medication alone.

## ADDITIONAL READING

1. Schatzberg AF and Nemeroff CB (Eds) (2004) *The American Psychiatric Press Textbook of Psychopharmacology*, 3rd edition, American Psychiatric Press, Washington, DC.
2. Greenhill LL, Shockey E, Halperin J, March J. (2003) Stimulants. In *Psychiatry*, 2nd edition (Eds Tasman A, Kay J, Lieberman JA), John Wiley & Sons, Ltd, London, 2062–2095.
3. MTA Cooperative Group (1999) 14 month randomized clinical trial of treatment strategies for children with attention deficit hyperactivity disorder. *Archives of General Psychiatry* **56** 1073–1086.
4. MTA Cooperative Group (2004) National Institute of Mental Health multimodal treatment study of ADHD follow-up: 24-month outcomes of treatment strategies for attention-deficit/hyperactivity disorder. *Pediatrics* **113**(4) 754–761.
5. Greenhill LL, Pliszka S, Dulcan MK, Bernet W, Arnold E, Beitchman J. (2002) Practice parameter for the use of stimulant medications in the treatment of children, adolescents, and adults. *Journal of the American Academy of Child and Adolescent Psychiatry* **41** 26S–49S.
6. Greenhill L. (2002) Childhood attention deficit hyperactivity disorder: pharmacological treatments. In *Treatments that Work*, 2nd edition (Eds Nathan PE, Gorman J), Saunders, Philadelphia, 25–55.

# 7

# COGNITIVE ENHANCERS AND TREATMENTS FOR ALZHEIMER'S DISEASE

## INTRODUCTION

By the late 1980s the advent and general acceptance of research-based diagnostic criteria for the dementia of Alzheimer's disease (AD), and an understanding of its underlying pathology along with mechanism-based pharmacological therapeutics, provided the framework for clinical trials to exploit a variety of new treatment strategies that might positively impact the illness. During the 1990s research- and consensus-based criteria were proposed to include vascular dementia, dementia with Lewy bodies, and frontotemporal dementia. These later criteria are evolving and have not been well-accepted and thus clinical trials including these populations have been limited.

## PHARMACOLOGY

### Mechanism of Action

Acetylcholine is inactivated when it is hydrolyzed to choline and acetate by acetylcholinesterase (AChE) and butyrylcholinesterase (BChE). By inhibiting the actions of

*Handbook of Psychiatric Drugs*   Jeffrey A. Lieberman and Allan Tasman
© 2006 John Wiley & Sons, Ltd

AChE, cholinesterase inhibitors (ChIs) effectively increase the amount of ACh available for intrasynaptic cholinergic receptor stimulation.

The ChIs differ among themselves in selectivity for AChE and BChE, mechanism of inhibition, competition with ACh for binding, and in pharmacokinetics. An unresolved question is whether or not these differences result in differential *clinical* efficacy, and different clinically observable adverse events. A summary of pharmacokinetics and pharmacodynamics is in Table 7-1.

- An acetylcholinesterase inhibitor can work at either of two sites on AChE, an ionic subsite or a catalytic esteratic subsite, to prevent the interaction between ACh and AChE. Tacrine and donepezil act at the ionic subsite; physostigmine and rivastigmine act at the catalytic esteratic subsite.
- Tacrine is an example of a non-selective inhibitor of AChE and BChE.
- Specific inhibition of AChE can occur with relatively little inhibition of when the side chains of the ChI interacts with the peripheral anionic site of AChE. Donepezil has this property and is therefore selective for AChE.
- Binding to the AChE sites may be either reversible or irreversible, and may be competitive or noncompetitive with acetylcholine. Galantamine is an example of a competitive ChI, competing with acetylcholine for AChE; tacrine is a non-competitive inhibitor.

In addition, AChE is present in a few molecular forms: one, a tetramer, G4, is located on the presynaptic membranes within the cholinergic synaptic cleft; another a monomer, G1, is found on postsynaptic membranes. Although G4 is decreased along with the neuronal loss of presynaptic cholinergic neurons, postsynaptic cholinergic receptor neurons and G1 ACh are not decreased significantly with AD or aging. Rivastigmine is a ChI that is highly selective for the postsynaptic G1 monomer form of AChE, while galantamine is less so, and donepezil is not selective.

L-glutamate is the main excitatory neurotransmitter in the central nervous system. Enhancement of its activity at the N-methyl-D-aspartate (NMDA) receptor may contribute to

■ TABLE 7-1. Pharmacodynamic and Pharmacokinetics of Marketed Cholinesterase Inhibitors

| DRUG | PHARMACODYNAMICS | ABSORPTION | BIOAVAIL-ABILITY | PEAK PLASMA (H) | ELIMINATION HALF-LIFE (H) | PROTEIN BINDING | METABOLISM/COMMENTS |
|---|---|---|---|---|---|---|---|
| Tacrine (Cognex) | Noncompetitive, reversible ChI, both butyryl and acetyl ChI, also multiple other actions | Delayed by food | 17% | 1–2 | 2–4 | 55% | Via 1A2, nonlinear pharmacokinetics; hepatoxicity requires regular monitoring of serum alamine aminotransferases. |
| Donepezil (Aricept) | Noncompetitive, reversible acetyl ChI. | Not affected by food | 100% | 3–4 | 70 | 96% | Via 2D6, 3A4. Nonlinear pharmacokinetics at 10 mg/d |
| Rivastigmine (Exelon) | Noncompetitive ChI, both butyryl and acetyl ChI may differentially affect different acetyl ChIs | Delayed by food | 40% | 1.4–2.6 | <5 | 40% | Hydrolysis by esterases and excreted in urine (nonhepatic). Duration of cholinesterase inhibition longer than plasma half-life. Nonlinear pharmacokinetics |
| Galantamine (Reminyl) | Competitive, reversible ChI, modulates nicotine receptors | Delayed by food | 90% | 1 | 7 | 18% | Via 2D6, 3A4 |

*Note:* Pharmacodynamic effects of some ChIs are longer than their elimination half-lives. Drugs that inhibit or induce the cytochrome enzymes above might be expected to increase or decrease blood levels. For the most part, however, drug interactions with donepezil, rivastigmine, and galantamine have not been clinical problems.

the pathogenesis of Alzheimer's disease, a phenomenon known as excitotoxicity. Memantine is a low affinity antagonist that is believed to reduce NMDA receptor overstimulation and restore receptor signaling function to more normal levels. It is also possible that reducing excitotoxicity may be neuroprotective by preventing neuronal calcium overload though there is no evidence that memantine modifies neurodegeneration in patients with Alzheimer's disease.

Several other strategies have been evaluated or may have potential as treatments for Alzheimer's disease (Table 7-2) though none are currently supported by adequate evidence of efficacy.

■ **TABLE 7-2.** Other Treatment Strategies

| DRUG | MECHANISM OF ACTION | EVIDENCE |
|------|---------------------|----------|
| Dopamine precursors/agonists (clonidine, guanefacine, amantadine, bromocriptine) | Enhance dopamine function | Studies suggest largely ineffective |
| Selegiline | MAO-B inhibitor | No adequate evidence of efficacy; see below for combination with vitamin E |
| Hydergine, nicergoline | Metabolic enhancement | No adequate evidence of efficacy |
| Nootropics (e.g., piracetam, oxiracetam) | Neuroprotection and cognitive enhancement | Non-specific effect on memory but no adequate evidence of efficacy in dementia |
| Neurotrophic factors (e.g., nerve growth factor) | May counteract atrophy of cholinergic neurones | Tested in small number of patients with limited success; no clinical trials |
| Estrogens | May enhance cognitive function and exert neurotrophic and neuroprotective effects | Epidemiological evidence suggests possible benefit but intervention studies show no efficacy |

| | | |
|---|---|---|
| NSAIDs | May reduce inflammation associated with neurodegeneration | Epidemiological evidence suggests possible benefit but intervention studies show no efficacy |
| Vitamin E (with selegiline), Ginkgo biloba | Antioxidants | Vitamin E plus selegiline maintains activities of daily living and prolongs survival in the community but without measurable improvement in cognitive test performance; Ginkgo biloba used in Europe for dementia syndromes but evidence for its cognitive enhancing properties is weak and inconsistent |
| Calcium channel blockers | Block increases intracellular calcium that may mediate cell death | May delay progression of memory impairment and onset of dementia but there is a lack of controlled data on efficacy |

## Pharmacokinetics

The cholinesterase inhibitors differ in their pharmacokinetic characteristics.

- Tacrine is poorly absorbed and has a short half-life. It is metabolized by CYP 1A2 hepatic enzymes.
- Donepezil has an oral bioavailability approaching 100%, with peak concentrations in four hours and linear pharmacokinetics. The drug accumulates at a constant rate, reaching steady state in about two weeks. Its relatively slow clearance, with a long half-life of 70 hours, enables once-daily administration, with little plasma level fluctuation. The drug is extensively bound to plasma proteins, including $\alpha_1$-acid glycoproteins. It is both excreted unchanged in the urine

and extensively metabolized by CYP 2D6 and 3A4 hepatic enzymes to active and inactive metabolites.

- The oral bioavailability of rivastigmine is about 40% up to a dose of 3 mg, after which AUC increases non-linearly. The peak plasma concentration occurs after one hour; maximum cholinesterase inhibition is about 60%, occurring after five hours and lasting for about ten hours. The elimination half-life is 1.5 hours. Rivastigmine undergoes hydrolysis by cholinesterase, with minimal hepatic involvement. It is excreted almost entirely in the urine as the sulfate conjugate of the decarbamylated metabolite.

- The oral bioavailability of galantamine is about 90%; peak serum concentrations occur after one hour after the immediate-release formulation, corresponding to the time of maximum inhibition of cholinesterase of 40%. The modified-release formulation is bioequivalent with the immediate-release tablet, though peak levels are both delayed (to 4.5–5 hours) and reduced (by 25%). The pharmacokinetics of galantamine are linear over the recommended dose range. It has low protein binding (18%) and 53% of the concentration in whole blood is distributed into red cells. It undergoes metabolism by CYP2D6 and CYP3A4 enzymes; about one-third of the dose is excreted unchanged in the urine and 12% as the glucuronide. Although total drug exposure (AUC) is increased by 35% in poor metabolizers, and by a similar amount in elderly patients, this is not clinically significant because the dose is titrated according to patient tolerability.

- Peak blood levels of memantine occur 3–7 hours after oral administration. It has low protein binding (45%) and a long half-life of 60–80 hours. Total exposure to the drug is 45% greater among women than men due to their lower body mass but the recommended dose is the same. Approximately half the dose of memantine is excreted unchanged in the urine; the remainder undergoes hepatic conversion to inactive metabolites. The metabolism of memantine is not affected by other drugs that induce or inhibit hepatic enzymes but drugs that alkalinize the urine (e.g., carbonic anhydrase inhibitors) reduce its clearance.

## INDICATIONS

The ChIs are approved for the treatment of mild to moderate Alzheimer's disease; memantine is currently the only agent approved for the treatment of moderate to severe Alzheimer's disease (defined as an MMSE score of less than 15).

Because of the actions of ChIs, these drugs require caution when used in patients with significant asthma, significant chronic obstructive pulmonary disease, cardiac conduction defects, or clinically significant bradycardia. Appropriate considerations are involved in general anesthesia as well since they may prolong the effects of succinylcholine-type drugs and memantine may increase the risk of adverse effects with ketamine.

## DRUG SELECTION

Approaches to the treatment of AD can be grouped into several conceptual categories (Table 7-3).

- One approach attempts to treat the behavioral symptoms such as agitation, aggression, psychosis, depression, anxiety, apathy, and sleep or appetite disturbances.
- A second approach attempts to treat the cognitive or neuropsychological signs of the illness such as memory, language, praxis, attention, orientation, and knowledge.
- A third approach attempts to slow the rate of progression of the illness, preserving patients' quality of life or autonomy. (Slowing the rate of decline might also be related to treating symptoms.)
- A fourth conceptual treatment approach is primary prevention, to delay the time to onset of illness. Success at this approach could have considerable impact: for example, delaying the onset of AD by five years would halve its incidence.

Thus far, only ChIs and memantine have shown generally consistent symptomatic efficacy in standardized, well-controlled multicenter trials lasting from six months to occasionally 12 months. Tacrine is associated with a relatively high risk of hepatotoxicity and is now little used.

■ **TABLE 7-3.** Conceptualized Treatment Strategies for Patients with Cognitive Impairment

---

Symptomatic and/or Restorative

Targets: impaired cognition, depression, psychosis, agitation, aggression, anxiety, insomnia

Examples: cholinesterase inhibitors, various cholinergic agonists, antidepressants, antipsychotics, mood stabilizers, antianxiety agents, hypnotics, NMDA and AMPA receptor modulators, angiotensin converting enzyme inhibitors

Neurotrophic factors: nerve growth factor, brain-derived neurotrophic factors, estrogens

Notes: some substances may have symptomatic or restorative effects but are unproven. These may include hydergine and neotropics such as piracetam.

Pathophysiologically-directed

Targets: underlying pathophysiology of neurodegeneration, including inflammation, production of oxidizing free radicals, excitatory amino acids.

Examples: anti-inflammatory agents, calcium channel blockers, NMDA and AMPA receptor modulators. Transplantation of hormonally active tissues, or NGF (nerve growth factor) gene therapy using viral vectors have been undertaken experimentally.

Etiologically-directed

Targets: β-amyloid formation or hyperphosphorylated tau protein.

Examples: modulators of APP expression, β- and γ-secretase inhibitors, inhibitors of beta-amyloid protein aggregation or deposition, immunization with antibodies to beta-amyloid.

Note: The interventions listed above include some that are available and marketed, as well as some that have not been demonstrated effective or safe, and some conceptual treatments not yet developed.

---

## TREATMENT INITIATION

The typical candidates for ChIs are as follows:

- Outpatients with AD of mild to moderate cognitive severity
- Those usually living at home or in an assisted living facility
- Those suffering from dementia as their main clinical problem
- Those in which behavioral syndromes such as psychosis, agitation, or significant insomnia, apathy, or depression do not dominate. ChIs can be given in the presence of most of these comorbid symptoms.

Treatment with cholinesterase inhibitors or memantine should be initiated at a low dose and, depending on tolerability, titrated to a target dose.

- Donepezil is initiated at 5 mg/day and then increased to 10 mg/day after four to six weeks. Raising the dose earlier increases the risk for cholinergic adverse events. The effective dose is 5–10 mg/day; the higher dose tends to be somewhat more effective when the various trials are evaluated as a group.
- The recommended starting dose of rivastigmine is 1.5 mg b.i.d., taken with meals. If this dose is well-tolerated after a minimum of two weeks of treatment, it may be increased to 3 mg b.i.d. Subsequent increases to 4.5 mg and then 6 mg b.i.d. should be based on good tolerability of the current dose and may be considered after a minimum of two weeks of treatment. Higher daily doses, averaging about 9 to 10 mg are associated with better efficacy than lower doses.
- The initial dose of galantamine is 4 mg b.i.d., and should be raised to 8 mg b.i.d. after two to four weeks. For patients who are tolerating medication but not responding, the dose can be raised to 12 mg b.i.d. after another four weeks.
- Treatment with memantine should be initiated at a dose of 5 mg/day and increased in increments of 5 mg at intervals of no less than one week to a target dose of 20 mg/day; doses greater than 5 mg/day should be divided into two and given in the morning and evening. Memantine is formulated as tablets and as a liquid that is administered by the carer via a syringe-like dosing device.

## Maintenance Treatment

Optimal duration of treatment with continuing efficacy is unknown but overall efficacy extends at least 9 to 12 months based on the clinical trials and open-label extension phases.

- It is not possible to predict individual patient responses to ChIs because of the great interpatient variability of response.
- Maintenance treatment can be continued as long as a therapeutic benefit for the patient seems apparent.

- The potential clinical benefit of ChIs should be reassessed on a regular basis.
- Discontinuation should be considered when evidence of a therapeutic effect is no longer present. However, there is consistent evidence from several studies that discontinuation usually leads to minimal to mild worsening on cognitive test scores, and the patient returns to the same level of cognitive impairment as the patient who took placebo all along in these clinical trials.

## Treatment Evaluation

Clinical experience suggests that ChIs may be effective at least for mildly disturbed behavior, and in delaying the onset of troublesome behaviors, perhaps by maintaining cognitive function or perhaps through enhancing attentional processes and activation. The evidence for this effect is based on incidental findings in cognitive enhancing studies and the symptoms that show the greatest improvement are depression and apathy.

It is difficult to assess individual patient response because of the variability of the deteriorating course of AD, and because most of the effect of medication is due to a stabilization or lack of worsening of symptoms or cognitive function while placebo-treated patients continue to decline. Therefore, the clinical observations of minimal or no clinical worsening may be sufficient reasons to continue medication treatment if patients are tolerating therapy.

Virtually all clinical trials of antidementia drugs undertaken in the US for regulatory purposes have used the Alzheimer's Disease Assessment Scale-cognitive subscale (ADAS-cog) as the index of cognitive change and the clinical global impression of change (CGI-C) as the "global" clinical measure. Secondary measures in AD clinical trials often include the Mini-Mental State Examination (MMSE), a brief, physician-administered, structured examination of cognitive function, and a variety of functional activity scales, such as the Alzheimer's Disease Cooperative Study-ADL (ADCS-ADL) Scale to assess aspects of daily functioning.

In clinical trials lasting up to six months, memantine has been shown to achieve small improvements in measures of

■ **TABLE 7-4.** FDA-Approved Drugs to Improve Cognitive Function in Alzheimer's Disease

| DRUG | HOW SUPPLIED | INITIAL DOSAGE | MAINTENANCE DOSAGE |
|------|-------------|----------------|--------------------|
| Tacrine | 10, 20, 30, and 40 mg capsules | 10 mg q.i.d. | 30 or 40 mg q.i.d. |
| Donepezil | 5 and 10 mg tablets | 5 mg q.i.d. | 5–10 mg q.i.d. |
| Rivastigmine | 1.5, 3, 4.5, and 6 mg capsules | 1.5 mg b.i.d. | 3, 4.5, or 6 mg b.i.d. |
| Galantamine | 4, 8, and 12 mg tablets, solution 4 mg/mL | 4 mg b.i.d. | 8 or 12 mg b.i.d. |
| Memantine | 5 and 10 mg tablets, oral solution 2 mg/mL | 5 mg q.i.d. | 10 mg b.i.d. |

Initial dosages should be maintained for at least 2 and preferably 4–6 weeks before increasing. Adverse events may occur with dosage titration.

cognition and activities of daily living and behavior. Patients had a clinically noticeable reduction in deterioration over this period with less functional and cognitive decline compared with placebo; they were also less likely to become agitated. Memantine also improves cognitive function, activities of daily living and behavior to a very small extent when added to established treatment with donepezil in patients with moderate to severe Alzheimer's disease.

## ADVERSE EFFECTS

### Cholinesterase Inhibitors

Most adverse events from ChIs are cholinergically mediated, and are characteristically mild in severity and short-lived, lasting only a few days (Table 7-5). Significant cholinergic side effects can occur in up to about 25% of patients receiving higher doses; often they are related to the rate of initial titration of medication.

Patients tend to become tolerant to the adverse events rapidly. However, anorexia and weight loss may be clinically significant problems over the longer term, especially in older, more medically ill, and nursing home patients, so these

■ **TABLE 7-5.** Adverse Effects of Cholinesterase Inhibitors

Summary of adverse event data in placebo-controlled, randomized clinical trials. The method of obtaining adverse events and their reporting vary among trials.

| *Drug* | *Adverse Events* |
|---|---|
| **Tacrine** | Nausea, vomiting, diarrhea, dyspepsia, myalgia, anorexia, dizziness, confusion, insomnia, rare agranulocytosis |
| | Approximately 50% of patients will develop direct, reversible hepatotoxicity manifested by elevated transaminases. |
| | Drug interactions may include increased cholinergic effects with bethanecol; increased plasma tacrine levels with cimetidine or fluvoxamine. This may occur by inhibition of P450 1A2. The association of tacrine with haloperidol may increase parkinsonism and tacrine increases theophylline concentration. |
| **Donepezil** | Nausea, diarrhea, insomnia, vomiting, muscle cramps, fatigue, anorexia, dizziness, abdominal pain, myasthenia, rhinitis, weight loss, anxiety, syncope (2 vs. 1%) |
| **Rivastigmine** | Nausea, vomiting, anorexia, dizziness, abdominal pain, diarrhea, malaise, fatigue, asthenia, headache, sweating, weight loss, somnolence, syncope (3 vs. 2%). Rarely, severe vomiting with esophageal rupture |
| **Galantamine** | Nausea, vomiting, diarrhea, anorexia, weight loss, abdominal pain, dizziness, tremor, syncope (2 vs. 1%) |

Adverse event estimates vary widely among the cholinesterase inhibitors from study to study and thus relative adverse event rates among drugs are difficult to estimate. Cholinergic side effects generally occur early and are related to initiating or increasing medication. They tend to be mild and self-limited. Medications should be restarted at lowest doses after temporarily stopping.

**General precautions with cholinesterase inhibitors** (as indicated in the prescribing information)

By increasing central and peripheral cholinergic stimulation cholinesterase inhibitors may:

1. increase gastric acid secretion, increasing the risk for GI bleeding especially in patients with ulcer disease or those taking anti-inflammatories
2. produce bradycardia, especially in patients with sick sinus or other supraventricular conduction delay, leading to syncope, falls, and possible injury
3. exacerbate obstructive pulmonary disease
4. cause urinary outflow obstruction
5. increase risk for seizures
6. prolong the effects of succinylcholine-type muscle relaxants

---

parameters should be monitored and medication reduced or discontinued to assess if appetite returns, if anorexia or weight loss become clinically significant.

Tacrine is poorly tolerated by 10–20% of patients and is associated with reversible hepatotoxicity. Transaminases may be elevated above three times the upper limit of normal in approximately 30% of patients within 6 to 12 weeks and reversed within 6 weeks of discontinuing medication. Although patients may be able to tolerate tacrine if it is reintroduced, it is now seldom prescribed.

Memantine appears to be relatively well-tolerated. Overall, the profile of reported adverse events is similar to that occurring in patients assigned to placebo and include dizziness, confusion, headache, hallucinations, tiredness; less commonly, vomiting, anxiety, hypertonia, cystitis, increased libido, and seizures have been reported. Some studies suggest a beneficial effect in reducing agitation but other studies do not show this effect.

## DRUG INTERACTIONS

- Inhibitors of CYP450 3A4 and 2D6 (such as ketoconazole and quinidine) and inducers of CYP 2D6 and CYP 3A4 (such as phenytoin, carbamazepine, dexamethasone, and phenobarbital) could either inhibit donepezil metabolism or increase the rate of elimination, but the clinical significance of this is not known.

- Rivastigmine's metabolism does not depend on liver P450 enzymes, and therefore no drug interactions related to the P450 system have been observed.
- Inhibitors of CYP3A4 or CYP2D6 may increase total exposure to galantamine; examples include paroxetine, fluoxetine, fluvoxamine, amitriptyline, cimetidine, and quinidine. The clinical significance of these interactions is uncertain but changes to concomitant drug therapy during treatment may result in a loss of efficacy or an increased risk of adverse effects. Galantamine appears to have no effect on the metabolism of other hepatic substrates.
- Memantine does not inhibit or induce hepatic microsomal enzymes; because it is excreted in the urine predominantly as unchanged drug, it is unlikely to be affected by drugs that affect hepatic enzyme function. Drugs that alkalinize the urine may reduce renal excretion of memantine and increase the risk of adverse effects. Memantine may increase the risk of central nervous system toxicity if administered with amantadine or dextromethorphan.

## SUMMARY

ChIs and memantine are the best proven efficacious symptomatic treatments for AD. They provide consistent, but small, effects in many patients with mild to moderate dementia, and have become the current pharmacological standard of treatment. Other therapeutic approaches are not as well tested or as clearly efficacious. Therefore, ChIs are likely to be actively used clinically for at least the next several years. Memantine is the only treatment approved for moderate to severe AD.

However, therapeutic results of these treatments are usually modest, affecting a minority of patients. In trials with ChIs, patients assessed were usually outpatients with mild to moderately severe dementia and few concomitant medical illnesses. Duration of effect beyond one year and long-term safety are not known, except for the uncontrolled observations of patients who continue on these drugs after the controlled trial. It is essential to understand the broad magnitudes of effects and the range of clinical utility. It often takes time, experience, and further studies for clinicians to appreciate the overall effectiveness and utility of new drugs. Long-term trials of the cholinesterase inhibitors in patients with mild cognitive impairment will help define the extent and limits of their efficacy, as will trials in vascular dementia.

## ADDITIONAL READING

1. Kaduszkiewicz H et al: Cholinesterase inhibitors for patients with Alzheimer's disease: systematic review of randomised clinical trials. *BMJ* 2005; 331:321–327
2. Tasman A, Kay J, Lieberman JA (Eds): *Psychiatry*, 2nd edition, John Wiley & Sons, Ltd, London, 2003

# 8

# DRUGS FOR TREATING SUBSTANCE ABUSE DISORDERS

## INTRODUCTION

Disorders of substance abuse are one of the commonest of psychiatric illnesses. They often complicate other psychiatric disorders and, together with complications of their own, they may also present in general medical practice. Clinicians must therefore be prepared to consider such a diagnosis in all clinical settings. Substance abuse disorders fall within the competency of psychiatry because they involve distressing behavioral and psychological syndromes but their medical sequelae mean that close co-operation between psychiatrists and other clinicians is essential.

The following summary focuses on the pharmacological management of intoxication and overdose syndromes; withdrawal syndromes; relapse prevention; and the treatment of comorbidity in substance abusers. Non-pharmacological strategies are very important components of management and their effects are additive to those of drug treatment. However, the focus of this book is drug treatment and these strategies are not discussed in depth.

*Handbook of Psychiatric Drugs*   Jeffrey A. Lieberman and Allan Tasman
© 2006 John Wiley & Sons, Ltd

## SYNDROMES ASSOCIATED WITH INTOXICATION

An accurate diagnosis is of fundamental importance in the assessment of patients who may be intoxicated. A full history must be obtained in the awareness that progression to potentially fatal overdose or withdrawal syndromes may occur. The focus of physical examination should be the acute effects of intoxication (such as vital and neurologic signs) and chronic signs and symptoms associated with drug dependence (size of liver, evidence of venipuncture). Drug use within the previous 4–12 hours can be determined by analysis of blood and breath samples whereas urinalysis is useful for assessing substance use within the preceding 24–72 hours. Urinalysis is the preferred option (with the exception of determining alcohol use) though saliva testing is becoming more widely used. Immediate results can be obtained with urine testing kits suitable for use in an office or clinic.

### Alcohol Intoxication

Intoxication with alcohol is associated with:

- maladaptive mental state (increased aggression)
- neurologic signs such as incoordination, unsteady gait, slurred speech
- impaired attention and memory

Stupor, coma, and cardiovascular collapse occur at high blood levels of alcohol (400–800 mg/dL) but the threshold for such effects depends on individual tolerance.

The rate at which blood alcohol levels decline averages 15 mg/dL/hour. Overall, nonpharmacological management is preferred because it avoids the risk of interactions between drugs and alcohol. Lorazepam 1–2 mg orally may be effective in belligerent patients who cannot be managed by supportive limit setting. If, despite these measures, the patient's condition worsens over the next 1–2 hours, an intramuscular injection of haloperidol 5 mg can be safely given.

In patients with significant mental status changes or alterations in sensorium, clinicians should be alert to the possibility of other causes such as head trauma or metabolic disturbance (e.g., thiamine deficiency). Furthermore, intoxicated patients with a recent history of regular heavy use and likely physiologic dependence on alcohol may be at risk from serious alcohol withdrawal (seizures or delirium) as the blood level clears, particularly if there is a past history of such complications. In that case, clinicians should consider starting tapering doses of a long-acting benzodiazepine (e.g., chlordiazepoxide) as acute intoxication begins to clear (see the section on alcohol withdrawal on page 223).

## Sedative–Hypnotic Intoxication

Benzodiazepine intoxication can be associated with behavioral disinhibition, potentially resulting in hostile or aggressive behavior; this effect is most commonly seen in patients combining benzodiazepines with alcohol. Benzodiazepine use is also frequently observed in combination with cocaine or opioids. Although benzodiazepines alone do not strongly suppress respiration (and pure benzodiazepine overdoses do not usually produce respiratory arrest and death), benzodiazepines may augment the respiratory depressant effects of other drugs such as alcohol, barbiturates, or opioids.

Suspected benzodiazepine overdosage can be reversed with the benzodiazepine antagonist flumazenil, which should be administered intravenously, beginning with 0.2 mg slow push over 30 seconds, followed by increments of 0.3 mg or 0.5 mg if no response, with total dose not to exceed 3 mg to 5 mg. If no response is obtained at those total doses, then another cause of stupor or coma should be considered.

When barbiturates are taken in relatively low doses, intoxication can be indistinguishable from alcohol intoxication. Symptoms include incoordination, sluggishness, poor memory, slow speech, poor comprehension, distorted mood, poor attention span, faulty judgment, and emotional lability. Other potential symptoms include hostility, moroseness, argumentativeness, and occasionally paraniod and suicidal ideation. As with alcohol, clinicians should be alert to other causes of mental status changes, and for patients with recent regular use and physiologic dependence on sedative–hypnotics, particularly short-acting agents (e.g., alprazolam, lorazepam), serious withdrawal can ensue, and prophylactic treatment with taper of a long-acting agent should be considered (see the section on sedative–hypnotic withdrawal on page 230).

## Opiate Intoxication

Although mild opiate intoxication can be stimulating, severe intoxication causes a maladaptive mental state with symptoms such as apathy; this is associated with pupillary constriction (characteristically midpoint with meperidine) or dilation if the patient has anoxia from severe overdose, central nervous system depression, and respiratory depression. Meperidine, propoxyphene, or pentazocine have active metabolites that may cause seizures.

Severe opiate intoxication is a life-threatening condition because of the high likelihood of respiratory depression or arrest. Opiate overdose is a common cause of death, especially among teenagers and young adults, and is particularly likely among individuals with low levels of tolerance, including inexperienced users, or patients who have recently detoxified or been abstinent for a period of time. Death from opiate overdose is an underappreciated risk, and, just as one would assess risk of suicide in depressed patients, clinicians evaluating a patient presenting with opiate intoxication should evaluate the risk of overdose, including level of tolerance and past history of overdose episodes.

The presence of miosis and respiratory depression at presentation is an indication for immediate treatment. An intravenous dose of the pure opiate antagonist naloxone HCl 0.4–0.8 mg usually reverses opiate-induced respiratory and CNS depression in two minutes. The dose may be repeated every 2–3 min if previous dose was not effective. Response occurs in the majority of patients after up to four doses but larger doses may be needed in cases of intoxication by highly potent opiates such as fentanyl or long-acting agents such as methadone. Naloxone has a duration of action of 1–2 h, which is shorter than that of opiates. When a response has been achieved, a naloxine infusion should therefore be initiated (initial dose 0.4 mg/h) and maintained for a minimum of 12 h.

When using naloxone it is important to note that:

1. CNS depression in patients with opiate overdose may be due to other causes, particularly if standard doses of naloxone are not effective.

2. Naloxone may suddenly precipitate an opiate withdrawal syndrome and should therefore be administered cautiously. Patients with precipitated withdrawal may become suddenly anxious, irritable, or combative, and try to leave the emergency ward against advice; such patients should be treated supportively, and naloxone discontinued temporarily until symptoms clear, after which naloxone may need to be resumed in response to resumed intoxication and respiratory depression, especially in the presence of longer-acting agonists. Such patients should be prevented, if at all possible, from leaving the emergency ward or clinic, since respiratory depression may return quickly once the naloxone wears off, or the patients may seek out and take more opiates. If opiate withdrawal persists, treatment should be initiated (see below).

3. Naloxone may not reverse the effects of buprenorphine. This partial opiate agonist, long available in parenteral form for analgesia, is now marketed in sublingual form [brand names Suboxone (buprenorphine-naloxone) and Subutex (buprenorphine)] as an alternative to methadone for agonist maintenance treatment of opioid dependence. Buprenorphine by itself produces less respiratory depression than other full opiate agonists, even at high doses, but death from overdose has been associated with combinations of buprenorphine and benzodiazepines.

## Cocaine and Amphetamine Intoxication

The effects of cocaine, amphetamines, and similar stimulants are characterized by the following:

- maladaptive psychological or behavioral changes such as anxiety, paranoid delusions, and hallucinations
- physical signs such as hypertension, tachycardia, mydriasis, perspiration, psychomotor agitation, and dyskinesia

- mild intoxication may be associated with behavior similar to hypomania, such as increased activity, gregariousness, and talkativeness; or irritability, anxiety, or agitation
- severe effects include respiratory depression, cardiac arrhythmias, delirium, and seizures

The behavioral, psychologic, and physical effects of amphetamine are longer-lasting than those of cocaine, typically resolving within 24–48 h.

Intoxication by cocaine and other stimulants may therefore cause serious physical effects; neurologic and cardiac should always be assessed and a medical plan to manage emergencies (hypertension, arrhythmias, seizures) should be developed.

The behavioral and psychologic effects of stimulant intoxication should, if possible, be managed in a reassuring and straightforward manner in a quiet environment. Lorazepam 2 mg is often successful if drug treatment is necessary. In fact, benzodiazepines are preferred even for more severe behavioral disturbances such as psychosis because antipsychotic agents may complicate management by their cardiovascular effects (such as tachycardia) or neurological complications (hyperthermia, seizures). If behavior escalates despite treatment with a benzodiazepine, cautious use of a high-potency antipsychotic such as haloperidol 5 mg may be appropriate. The clearance of amphetamine is increased by acidification of the urine but this technique is not recommended in cases of cocaine intoxication.

## Intoxication by LSD, Mescaline, MDMA ('Ecstasy'), and Psilocybin

Intoxication by an hallucinogen is associated with:

- maladaptive psychologic effects (anxiety, paranoia, belief of going insane)
- changes of perception (perception becomes more intense, depersonalization, hallucinations, synesthesia)
- physical signs (mydriasis, tachycardia)

The usual treatment option is the oral administration of 20 mg of diazepam; this should attenuate the LSD experience and alleviate any associated panic to a halt within 20 min and is considered a superior treatment option than the once-common 'talking down' method.

'Flashback' (a transient perceptual abnormality reminiscent of a previous episode of intoxication by an hallucinogen) can be triggered by anxiety, fatigue or use of drugs such as cannabis. A flashback may be distressing, particularly if the original episode was distressing. These events are short-lived and usually remit spontaneously. Supportive reassurance is therefore usually sufficient but a benzodiazepine may be useful in carefully selected patients who experience anticipatory anxiety.

MDMA ('Ecstasy') is reported to produce increased feelings of well-being, interpersonal warmth, and connectedness, and the drug is often taken in social situations including large gatherings ('raves'). Hyperthermia and occasional deaths have been reported, perhaps abetted by overactivity and dehydration.

## Phencyclidine Intoxication

Intoxication by phencyclidine (PCP) is associated with:

- maladaptive changes in behavior, such as belligerence, assaultiveness, and impulsivity
- physical signs such as nystagmus, hypertension, ataxia, muscle rigidity, diminished responsiveness to pain, seizures, and coma
- lower doses typically cause excitation whereas higher doses are dangerously sedative

The duration of symptoms of intoxication varies: PCP undergoes enterohepatic recirculation, resulting in symptom recurrence after a period of quiescence. Patients should therefore be observed for 12 h before they are discharged.

Interventions other than drug treatment include a quiet environment and close observation for the behavioral and physical effects of intoxication. 'Talking down' is reportedly less useful than in the management of hallucination intoxication. Patients may have a diminished response to pain (PCP has anesthetic activity) and if they become belligerent they may struggle violently against restraint. In such cases there is a risk of rhabdomyolysis and patients should be closely monitored.

When pharmacologic agents are used to treat PCP intoxication, the aim is usually to produce sedation or relieve psychosis; no useful PCP-receptor antagonist has been developed. For general sedation, a benzodiazepine such as lorazepam may be used orally or intramuscularly. Haloperidol is a reasonable neuroleptic agent when psychotic agitation is unresponsive to benzodiazepines. More anticholinergic neuroleptics may act to enhance the anticholinergic properties of PCP itself. If neuroleptics are used, one must remember that PCP itself can produce muscle rigidity and acute dystonias. Urinary acidification has been recommended to increase the excretion of PCP in the urine. However, this may also exacerbate a developing metabolic acidosis and increase the risk of renal failure resulting from rhabdomyolysis.

The aim of drug treatment is to relieve symptoms through sedation and reduce psychosis. There is no specific antagonist for PCP. A benzodiazepine such as lorazepam (oral or intramuscular) is preferred for general sedation; in cases where psychotic agitation does not respond to a benzodiazepine, haloperidol is a reasonable choice. There is a risk that some antipsychotic agents may worsen some of the effects of PCP, which has anticholinergic activity and may cause muscle rigidity and acute dystonias.

## DRUG TREATMENT OF WITHDRAWAL SYNDROMES

Some general principles are important when considering pharmacologic treatments for particular withdrawal syndromes:

When monitoring treatment:

- set clear targets
- make serial assessments and modify on the basis of these assessments

Psychosocial factors:

- prepare the patient
- place emphasis on detoxification as a beginning to treatment

From a pharmacologic standpoint, an ideal agent for the treatment of withdrawal should have the following characteristics:

- efficacy in relieving the complete range of abstinence signs and symptoms for a given type of withdrawal
- a relatively long duration of action and gradual offset of effects
- a high degree of safety in the dosage needed to suppress withdrawal (i.e., high therapeutic index)
- it should be available by a variety of routes of administration and have little abuse potential in itself

Some equally general important aspects that may be overlooked include:

- keep clear treatment targets in mind
- consider structured rating scales for measuring symptom severity
- treatment must be guided by serial assessment of the clinical response: protocols offer useful guidance but orders must be reviewed and rewritten, frequently daily. It is dangerous to detoxify a patient on autopilot

From the patient's perspective:

- they should be told what to expect from the experience of detoxication
- physicians should make the effort to engage them in a joint effort to alleviate symptoms safely
- they should be awarae that they are unlikely to be free of distress
- it may be possible to accomplish detoxication on an outpatient basis for those who have relatively good health and sufficient social stability
- most importantly, they must understand that detoxication is the beginning of treatment of their chronic problems with substance dependence – it is not, by itself, a treatment for addiction

## Alcohol Withdrawal

Alcohol withdrawal symptoms typically occur 6–12 h after the end of, or a reduction in, heavy and prolonged drinking;

they may also occur despite the presence of significant blood alcohol levels if those levels are falling.

Alcohol withdrawal symptoms include:

- autonomic hyperactivity
- increased muscle tremor (may affect the hand, eyelids, or tongue)
- insomnia
- nausea or vomiting
- transient hallucinations or illusions
- agitation
- anxiety

The alcohol withdrawal syndrome also includes generalized seizures. These may occur 12–48 h after the end of alcohol consumption; they are typically nonfocal and confined to one or two episodes.

Alcohol withdrawal delirium (delirium tremens) usually occurs 3–5 days after the end of consumption. This is associated with:

- disturbance of consciousness
- change in cognition
- perceptual disturbance
- agitation, belligerence, and elevation in vital signs may also occur

This delirium is more likely to occur in the presence of a comorbid physical disorder or in someone with a history of seizures or delirium during previous withdrawal syndromes. The occurrence of delirium is therefore an indication for reassessing the patient's medical status to identify possibly undiagnosed illness. Alcohol withdrawal is a medical emergency and can be life threatening without appropriate supportive medical treatment.

Appropriate management greatly reduces the risk that uncomplicated withdrawal will progress to seizures or delirium. Patients should undergo systematic assessment when they begin detoxication and during the process. The Clinical Institute Withdrawal Assessment for alcohol scale is a simple tool that is widely used (Table 8-1).

■ **TABLE 8-1.** Clinical Institute Withdrawal Assessment for Alcohol Scale*

---

Patient: _____

Time: ____: ____

(24 hour clock, midnight = 00:00)

Date: ___ /___ /___

      y  m  d

**NAUSEA AND VOMITING:** Ask, "Do you feel sick to your stomach? Have you vomited?" Observation.

0—no nausea and no vomiting

1—mild nausea with no vomiting

2

3

4—intermittent nausea with dry heaves

5

6

7—constant nausea, frequent dry heaves and vomiting

**TREMOR:** Arms extended and fingers spread apart. Observation.

0—no tremor

1—not visible, but can be felt fingertip to fingertip

2

3

4—moderate, with patient's arms extended

5

6

7—severe, even with arms not extended

**PAROXYSMAL SWEATS:** Observation.

0—no sweat visible

1—barely perceptible sweating, palms moist

2

3

4—beads of sweat obvious on forehead

5

6

7—drenching sweats

Pulse or heart rate, taken for

1 minute: _____

Blood pressure: ____ /____

**TACTILE DISTURBANCES:** Ask, "Have you any itching, pins-and-needles sensations, any burning, any numbness, or do you feel bugs crawling on or under your skin?" Observation.

0—none

1—very mild itching, pins and needles, burning, or numbness

■ **TABLE 8-1.** (Continued)

2—mild itching, pins and needles, burning, or numbness
3—moderate itching, pins and needles, burning, or numbness
4—moderately severe hallucinations
5—severe hallucinations
6—extremely severe hallucinations
7—continuous hallucinations

**AUDITORY DISTURBANCES:** Ask, "Are you more aware of sounds around you? Are they harsh? Do they frighten you? Are you hearing anything that is disturbing to you? Are you hearing things that you know aren't there?" Observation.

0—not present
1—very mild harshness or ability to frighten
2—mild harshness or ability to frighten
3—moderate harshness or ability to frighten
4—moderately severe hallucinations
5—severe hallucinations
6—extremely severe hallucinations
7—continuous hallucinations

**VISUAL DISTURBANCES:** Ask, "Does the light appear to be too bright? Is its color different? Does it hurt your eyes? Are you seeing anything that is disturbing you? Are you seeing things that you know aren't there?" Observation.

0—not present
1—very mild sensitivity
2—mild sensitivity
3—moderate sensitivity
4—moderately severe hallucinations
5—severe hallucinations
6—extremely severe hallucinations
7—continuous hallucinations

**ANXIETY:** Ask, "Do you feel nervous?" Observation.

0—no anxiety, at ease
1—mildly anxious
2
3
4—moderately anxious, or guarded, so anxiety is inferred
5
6
7—equivalent to acute panic states as seen in severe delirium or acute schizophrenic reactions

**AGITATION:** Observation.

0—normal activity
1—somewhat more than normal activity

2

3

4—moderately fidgety and restless

5

6

7—paces back and forth during most of the interview, or constantly thrashes about

**HEADACHE, FULLNESS IN HEAD:** Ask, "Does your head feel different? Does it feel like there is a band around your head?" Do not rate dizziness or lightheadedness. Otherwise, rate severity.

0—not present

1—very mild

2—mild

3—moderate

4—moderately severe

5—severe

6—very severe

7—extremely severe

**ORIENTATION AND CLOUDING OF SENSORIUM:** Ask, "What day is this? Where are you? Who am I?"

0—oriented and can do serial additions

1—cannot do serial additions or is uncertain about date

2—disoriented for date by no more than 2 calendar days

3—disoriented for date by more than 2 calendar days

4—disoriented for place and/or person

Total CIWA-A score ____

Rater's initials ____

Maximum possible score—67

---

* This scale is not copyrighted and may be used freely.

See Sullivan JT, Sykora K, Schneiderman J, Narango CA, Sellers EM (1989). Assessment of alcohol withdrawal: the revised Clinical Institute Withdrawal Instrument for Alcohol Scale (CIWA-AR). *British Journal of Addiction* 84:1353–1357.

The scale should be administered at regular intervals (initially every 1–2 h) 6–24 h after the patient's last drink until there are at least two consecutive assessments with scores less than 8–10; structured assessment can then safely end. Closer monitoring is indicated if the score exceeds 15; the interpretation of intermediate scores depends on clinical judgment, taking into account issues such as the history of withdrawal episodes and the degree of discomfort experienced by the patient.

Provided serial clinical assessments are carried out, it is relatively straightforward to strike a balance between withdrawal and intoxication. The most common error associated with drug treatment of withdrawal is prescribing doses that are too small or dose intervals that are too long.

Benzodiazepines are the treatment of choice for alcohol withdrawal. They are relatively safe compared with other sedative–hypnotic drugs; and they reduce the frrequency of seizures and delirium. Alcoholics are cross-tolerant to their effects and may therefore require doses that would be considered high for non-tolerant individuals.

The benzodiazepines can be dividied into two classes according to their duration of action:

- *Longer-acting agents* include chlordiazepoxide (which has lower abuse potential and may therefore be preferred) and diazepam. These agents undergo both oxidation and glucuronidation. It is an advantage that blood levels of these agents decline gradually during the tapering process because this is associated with greater between-dose patient comfort and possibly better seizure prophylaxis. The disadvantage is that if elimination is delayed (for example, in elderly patients or patients with impaired liver or pulmonary function), there is a risk that accumulation will cause toxicity.
- *Shorter-acting agents* include oxazepam and lorazepam, which undergo only glucuronidation. Their advantage is that they are well metabolized and eliminated by elderly people, with less chance of accumulation and toxicity in patients with liver disease. The disadvantage is that between-dose blood levels may decline abruptly, increasing the risk of breakthrough symptoms and seizures.

All may be administered orally or intravenously; only lorazepam is available as an intramuscular injection.

The patient's response should be determined by serial assessments and drug treatment should be adjusted according to clinical need. For example, increasing signs of withdrawal indicate the need for an increase in dose or a decrease in the dose interval. A degree of sedation is desirable but if over-sedation occurs drug treatment should be withheld until it is again clinically indicated. Recommendations for medication are summarized in Figure 8-1.

Hallucinations that develop during delirium are relatively refractory to benzodiazepines alone; if they occur despite substitution therapy with a sedative–hypnotic, adjunctive haloperidol 2–5 mg may be administered.

If persistent tachycardia or hypertension occur the possibility should be excluded that they may be due to inadequately treated withdrawal. Treatment with a beta-blocker or clonidine has been successful; these agents may also decrease vital signs and tremor but they do not prevent seizures.

As an alternative management strategy, a patient attending for detoxication may be 'frontloaded' with 1–2 hourly doses of diazepam or chlordiazepoxide to achieve sedation. Because

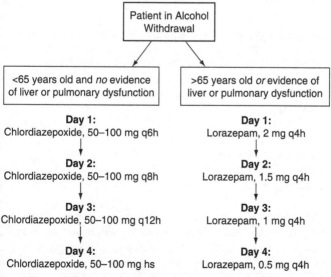

**FIGURE 8-1.** Medication recommendations for treating alcohol withdrawal. From Selzer J (2000). Drugs for Treating Substance Abuse. In *Psychiatric Drugs*, Lieberman JA and Tasman A (eds.) WB Saunders, pp. 214–241. © 2000, with permission from Elsevier.

these drugs have a long elimination half-life, their effects diminish slowly over the period of withdrawal. However, the need remains for careful serial assessment while there is a risk of withdrawal complications.

Reports of experience with carbamazepine and valproate in the treatment of alcohol withdrawal are promising and they may have a role in special circumstances. However, the safety and efficacy of benzodiazepines is currently unsurpassed.

Thiamine is indicated for every patient with alcoholism to prevent Wernicke's encephalopathy and Korsakoff's amnestic syndrome. The typical dose is 100 mg/day; replacement with thiamine should begin immediately and must precede administration of intravenous glucose. Nutritional management is completed with the addition of folate and multivitamin supplements, though the need is less acute. Although some believe that magnesium supplementation prevents withdrawal seizures, there is no consensus on its role in the absence of proven magnesium deficiency.

## Withdrawal from Sedative–Hypnotics

Symptoms of sedative–hypnotic withdrawal include:

- tremor
- anxiety
- insomnia
- anorexia
- nausea and vomiting
- postural hypotension
- seizures

These symptoms are qualitatively similar to those of alcohol withdrawal and the Clinical Institute withdrawal assessment scale is therefore useful to document symptom progression and the response to treatment. Withdrawal from sedative–hypnotic drugs is a medical emergency: if untreated there is a risk of serious complications (such as hyperpyrexia) and death. The nature of withdrawal symptoms is similar for all sedative–hypnotics but the rate of onset and decline depends on the half-life of individual drugs. For short-acting agents (e.g., seco-barbital), withdrawal symptoms begin 12–24 h after the last dose. By contrast, symptoms develop more slowly for long-acting agents (e.g., diazepam) and may become maximal one week after the last dose.

Similar to the treatment for alcohol withdrawal, benzodi-azepine taper (as described above) is a good choice, particu-larly if the patient is dependent on benzodiazepines.

An excellent alternative for substitution therapy in sedative–hypnotic withdrawal is phenobarbital. This long-acting agent is associated with low between-dose fluctuation in blood levels; it has low potential for abuse and a wide margin between therapeutic and lethal blood levels. The symptoms of phenobarbital intoxication (ataxia, slurred speech, nystagmus) are readily apparent and easy to respond to in a detoxication protocol.

In detoxication of sedative–hypnotic dependency, the first step is to obtain a history of drug use. This enables the physi-cian to estimate the dose of phenobarbital equivalent to the total dose of sedative–hypnotic, as specified in Table 8-2.

The total phenobarbital equivalent dose is then summed and divided into a three-times daily dose regimen. The total daily dose of phenobarbital rarely exceeds 500 mg even for patients with extreme dependence.

In the event that acute withdrawal symptoms emerge before substitution therapy has begun, the first dose of phenobarbital may be administered by intramuscular injection. Withdrawal or intoxication symptoms should then be reassessed 1–2 h later to determine the next dose of phenobarbital.

The degree of dependence can be assessed by serial admin-istration of pentobarbital 200 mg but it is not clear whether this approach is superior to direct substitution with phenobarbital, which is speedy, simple, and safe.

There should be no signs of sedative–hypnotic withdrawal or phenobarbital toxicity 24–48 h after beginning substitution therapy with phenobarbital and the dose reduction phase may then begin. This involves a reduction in phenobarbital dose of 30 mg/day, maintaining the three times daily dose regimen. If phenobarbital toxicity occurs (slurred speech, nystagmus, ataxia), the next dose should be withheld and the total daily

■ **TABLE 8-2.** *Phe*nobarbital Withdrawal Equivalents of Sedative–Hypnotics

| CLASS/GENERIC NAME | DOSE (mg)* |
|---|---|
| **BENZODIAZEPINES** | |
| Alprazolam | 1 |
| Chlordiazepoxide | 25 |
| Clonazepam | 2 |
| Clorazepate | 7.5 |
| Diazepam | 10 |
| Estazolam | 1 |
| Flurazepam | 15 |
| Halazepam | 40 |
| Lorazepam | 2 |
| Oxazepam | 10 |
| Prazepam | 10 |
| Quazepam | 15 |
| Temazepam | 15 |
| Triazolam | 0.25 |
| **BARBITURATES** | |
| Amobarbital | 100 |
| Butabarbital | 100 |
| Butalbital | 100 |
| Pentobarbital | 100 |
| Secobarbital | 100 |
| **OTHER** | |
| Chloral hydrate | 500 |
| Ethchlorvynol | 500 |
| Glutethimide | 250 |
| Meprobamate | 1200 |
| Methyprylon | 200 |
| Zolpidem | 5 |

* Dose equivalent to 30 mg of phenobarbital for withdrawal.

Adapted from Wesson DR, Smith DE, Ling W, Seymour RB: Chapter 17: Sedative-Hypnotics. In: Lowinson JH, Ruiz P, Millman RB, Langrod JG, editors: *Substance Abuse: A Comprehensive Textbook*, 4th ed. Philadelphia: Lippincott Williams and Wilkins; 2005.

dose should be reduced. In the event of objective signs of withdrawal, the daily dose of phenobarbital is increased and the dose reduction phase is delayed until the patient is stabilized again.

# Withdrawal from Opiates

Opiate withdrawal, by contrast with withdrawal from sedative–hypnotics, may be intensely uncomfortable but for most adults (with the important exceptions of adults with little reserve, such as those with advanced AIDS, and newborn infants) it is not usually life-threatening. Nevertheless, easing symptoms can be an important part of the process of engaging an individual in treatment for their opiate addiction and to facilitate other medical treatment.

The time to onset of withdrawal symptoms depends on the duration of action of the opiate. Symptoms typically begin 6–24 h after the last dose of a short-acting agent such as heroin but 48–72 h after longer-acting opiates like methadone. The administration of an opiate antagonist (e.g., naloxone) can precipitate severe withdrawal symptoms, including: dysphoria, nausea and vomiting, muscle aches, lacrimation or rhinorrhea, dilated pupils, piloerection, diarrhea, diaphoresis, yawning, fever, and insomnia.

Methadone is approved by the FDA for the treatment of opiate withdrawal. Regulations for its use differ between states but they typically allow its use for inpatient detoxication and methadone maintenance. Its use in an outpatient setting for the management of opiate withdrawal is not permitted except as part of a licensed methadone maintenance treatment program.

Oral methadone has a long duration of action. The initial dose of 15–20 mg is given when signs of opiate withdrawal (not simply reports of drug craving) are evident. An additional 5–10 mg may be given 1–2 h later if symptoms persist or worsen. A dose of 40 mg/day usually controls signs of withdrawal well (note that the dose for the different indication of long-term methadone maintenance may often be higher). When oral administration is impossible due to withdrawal symptoms, methadone 5 mg may be administered as an intramuscular injection. Having reached a dose that relieves withdrawal symptoms, the daily dose can be tapered by a gradual 10–20% for full detoxication.

A newly available option for treatment of opioid withdrawal is the schedule III opioid partial agonist buprenorphine, which is now available for use in office-based practice by any physician who has taken a brief training and certification. Although the use of schedule II drugs such as methadone for the treatment of opiate dependence is restricted to hospitals or specially licensed clinics (leading to a shortage of facilities where opiate-dependent individuals can receive appropriate treatment), the Drug Addiction Treatment Act of 2000 introduced less stringent regulations, allowing the use of narcotic drugs for the treatment of addiction in the office or any other health-care setting by any licensed physician who has taken a brief training course and obtained registration, thereby increasing access to treatment. Two new formulations of buprenorphine (Subutex and Suboxone sublingual tablets) were the first products to be approved by the FDA under this Act for the treatment of opioid dependence. Subutex contains only buprenorphine in doses of 2–8 mg; Suboxone also contains the opioid antagonist naloxone (0.5 and 2 mg respectively); the purpose of the naloxone is to discourage diversion of the medication for abuse intravenously (crushing the pills and injecting them), since naloxone is poorly absorbed after oral or sublingual administration, but if injected it would produce precipitated withdrawal.

Buprenorphine is an excellent detoxification agent because of its long duration of action owing to very high affinity for and very slow dissociation from opioid receptors. Starting buprenorphine must be done carefully, because of the partial agonism. If administered too close in time to the last dose of a full agonist such as heroin, buprenorphine will precipitate withdrawal, and the withdrawal produced can be atypical and in rare cases has been observed to include delirium. Precipitated withdrawal is more likely among patients dependent on long-acting agonists (e.g., methadone) or high daily doses of a shorter-acting agonist such as heroin. Thus, when starting buprenorphine, the clinician should wait for symptoms of opioid withdrawal to begin to appear before giving the first dose of buprenorphine, which should be a test dose of 2 mg [Subutex 2 mg, or Suboxone (2 mg buprenorphine/0.5 mg naloxone)]. If this dose is well tolerated, administer another 2 mg 1 h later, and up to 8 mg total on the first day, and up to 16 mg on the second day. After this, buprenorphine can be tapered slowly to zero over 10 days to 2 weeks. Considerable flexibility in the taper schedule is possible, including a much faster taper, since the slow dissociation from receptors in itself effectively produces a taper. However, clinicians should also be alert for the emergence of low-grade withdrawal symptoms (fatigue, anxiety, mild flu-like physical symptoms) in the weeks after discontinuing buprenorphine. This subacute or protracted withdrawal can be observed from any opioid drug but can seem surprising with buprenorphine because the taper phase of a buprenorphine detoxification is usually comfortable and uneventful.

If one of the first few doses of buprenorphine administered is followed by a rapid worsening of withdrawal symptoms, this is precipitated withdrawal, and no further buprenorphine should be given; at this point it is probably best to treat with a full agonist (methadone), although one could also wait for precipitated withdrawal to clear and full-blown opiate withdrawal (from whatever the patient was addicted to) to emerge, after which one can try again beginning with a test dose of 2 mg buprenorphine.

A number of nonnarcotic medications are useful in treating the symptoms of opiate withdrawal. These include the α-adrenergic receptor agonist and antihypertensive clonidine, which is particularly helpful with the autonomic symptoms of withdrawal as well as the anxiety, benzodiazepines (clonazepam is typically used), which are particularly helpful for anxiety and insomnia, antiemetics, and NSAIDs for muscle aches (oral agents such as ibuprofen, or toradol which can be given parenterally). Although with clonidine alone the autonomic symptoms may be well controlled, patients often complain of greater subjective distress with clonidine than with an agonist such as methadone or buprenorphine.

Clonidine is used to assist detoxication in individuals using illegal opiates in circmstances where methadone is not permitted (e.g., outpatient settings) and to relieve abstinence symptoms in a patient stopping methadone maintenance. In clonidine-assisted detoxication, the main side effects are hypotension, which may cause doses to be withheld or treatment discontinued, and sedation. Hypotension may be worsened by diarrhea or vomiting, which are common in opiate withdrawal. Patients should be encouraged to take plenty of fluids, and sports drinks such as Gatorade are particularly helpful because they also supply electrolytes. Because clonidine by itself does not treat all aspects of withdrawal, clonidine is most effective in combination with the other agents mentioned above. A protocol for clonidine-assisted detoxication is given in Table 8-3.

A combination of clonidine with naltrexone has been used to achieve a more rapid withdrawal followed by maintenance with naltrexone. This strategy requires close monitoring of the patient and an experienced clinician to titrate the dose of clonidine against naltrexone-induced withdrawal symptoms. The acceptability of maintenance therapy with naltrexone to opiate addicts is disappointing.

With opiate detoxification, it is particularly important to consider the indications for it, and to establish an adequate treatment plan after detoxification is completed. Chronic opioid use induces tolerance, and detoxification reduces or eliminates tolerance. Because of the loss of tolerance,

■ TABLE 8-3. Clonidine Detoxification

| DAY | SHORT-ACTING OPIATE* | LONG-ACTING OPIATE† |
|---|---|---|
| Day 1 | 0.1 mg q4h | 0.1 mg q4h |
| Days 2–4 | 0.1–0.2 mg q4h (depending on symptoms) | 0.1–0.2 mg q4h (depending on symptoms) |
| Days 5–10 | Reduce daily dose by 0.2–0.4 mg/d | Maintain on 0.4–1.2 mg/d |
| Day 11 | | Reduce daily dose by 0.2–0.4 mg/d |

Adjunctive medication: oxazepam (in limited supplies) for sleep or agitation; ibuprofen or toradol for muscle or bone pain; bismuth subsalicylate for diarrhea; prochlorperazine or odansetron for nausea.

* For example, heroin.
† For example, methadone.
From Selzer J (2000). Drugs for Treating Substance Abuse. In *Psychiatric Drugs*, Lieberman JA and Tasman A (eds.) WB Saunders, pp. 214–241. © 2000, with permission from Elsevier.

detoxified opiate addicts are at increased risk of death from opiate overdose; doses that they routinely self-administered previously when tolerant could now be lethal, a problem exacerbated by the variable and sometimes high potency of illicit heroin. In general, the risk of relapse following opioid detoxification is high. Therefore, patients should be assessed for overdose risk, and those with a history of past overdoses, or with multiple past relapses, should be encouraged to take agonist maintenance treatment, with methadone or buprenorphine, rather than undergoing detoxification. For those not entering agonist maintenance, a strong plan for psychosocial treatment is important, for example long-term residential treatment or therapeutic community, a good outpatient treatment program, supplemented by a self-help group (Alcoholics Anonymous, or Narcotics Anonymous).

## Management of Withdrawal in Patients with Multiple Dependencies

Patients may have dependencies on drugs from more than one pharmacological class. It is safest first to suppress each of the abstinence syndromes then attempt detoxication from the most dangerous class of drugs first. In patients who are dependent on both opiates and sedative–hypnotics or alcohol, withdrawal from a sedative–hypnotic or alcohol may cause convulsions or death and is clearly more important than opiate withdrawal, which is associated with discomfort. In such cases, a steady dose of methadone or buprenorphine should be maintained while detoxication from sedative–hypnotics or alcohol is achieved; methadone detoxication may then proceed.

## AGENTS TO AID RELAPSE PREVENTION

The emergence of treatments to prevent post-detoxication relapse in patients with dependency is an exciting development in psychopharmacology. A wide variety of strategies has been developed:

- aversive therapy depends on creating a biochemical environment in which the effect of a substance is unpleasant rather than gratifying

- antagonist therapy blocks the gratifying effect of a substance (without replacing it with an aversive one)
- agonist therapy involves substituting a drug of abuse for a medicine which acts at the same receptor but has safer pharmacological properties
- less widely used, medications may be used to correct the putative neurochemical changes associated with drug abuse
- new agents are being developed that act at the neurophysiological steps intermediate between the use and effect of abused substances, such as synaptic transporters

There is evidence that psychosocial interventions increase the effectiveness of drug treatment and psychopharmacological strategies for relapse prevention are not intended to replace them. In patients who receive intensive psychosocial interventions that are relevant to drug dependency problems, the incremental benefit of adding medication to prevent relapse prevention is reduced. On the other hand, a psychosocial treatment tailored to take advantage of the effect of the medication may synergize to produce a stronger effect. The physician may sometimes be expected to justify—to both the patient and other clinicians—substituting one drug for another as part of the treatment for drug dependence. The argument rests on the clear difference between taking medication prescribed by a physician and using drugs of abuse to which the patient is addicted.

## Medications for Alcohol Dependence

Three medications are now FDA approved for treatment of alcohol dependence: disulfiram, naltrexone, and acamprosate.

Disulfiram binds irreversibly to aldehyde dehydrogenase, the enzyme that catalyzes the oxidation of acetaldehyde (a metabolite of alcohol) to acetic acid. It therefore changes the body's response to alcohol. Ingestion of alcohol results in the accumulation of acetaldehyde, causing an extremely dysphoric experience of palpitations, hypotension, nausea and vomiting, and diaphoresis. This is self-limiting but it can produce substantial stress to the cardiovascular system, particularly with high doses both of alcohol and of disulfiram. This is generally not dangerous in young, healthy individuals, but could lead to cardiovascular collapse and death in patients with significant cardiovascular or renal disease. Disulfiram has also been associated with liver toxicity, and education of the patient about signs of liver failure and periodic monitoring of liver functions are advisable.

When the FDA approved disulfiram as a treatment for alcoholism, standards for efficacy studies were lower than they are today. The best evidence suggests that, although disulfiram is associated with a reduction in the number of drinking days in alcoholics who drink while taking it, compliance with medication, not the effects of disulfiram, is probably important for a better outcome.

In the view of many clinicians, disulfiram may nonetheless provide an important disincentive to drink in well-motivated patients. There is evidence that using disulfiram as part of a contract involving the spouse offers the prospect of good results: the alcoholic agrees to allow the spouse to witness disulfiram ingestion and the spouse agrees to refrain from comment on the alcoholic's drinking. If disulfiram is taken regularly, it will prevent drinking, since even a small amount of intake will make the patient sick.

The usual dose of disulfiram is 250 mg/day; this maintains inhibition of acetaldehyde dehydrogenase while minimizing side effects such as lethargy. Some patients will report being able to drink without consequence on 250 mg per day. This may simply mean the patient is not actually taking the medication regularly, and should prompt gentle inquiry into compliance. However, some patients do need higher doses, up to 500 mg per day. In rare cases, drug-induced psychosis may occur due to inhibition of dopamine α-hydroxylase by disulfiram. There is also a risk of interactions between disulfiram and medications (e.g., tricyclic antidepressant and phenytoin levels are increased). Patients should be made aware that alcohol is a component of products other than beverages (e.g., shaving lotions). Significant inhibition of acetaldehyde dehydrogenase, and therefore the risk of reactions if alcohol is ingested, lasts for up to two weeks after stopping disulfiram.

It is believed that the reinforcing effects of alcohol may be mediated by endogenous opiate systems and this hypothesis underlies the use of naltrexone in alcohol relapse prevention.

Naltrexone combined with structured psychosocial treatment has been associated with improvements in complete abstinence, less craving for alcohol when the patient was abstinent, and less drinking once drinking began. Psychosocial treatments that have proven particularly effective in combination with naltrexone are those, such as cognitive behavioral relapse prevention, that emphasize coping skills for handling various sources of relapse risk. The recommended dose is 50 mg per day. This agent differs from disulfiram in that there is no added ill effect once drinking begins. It may limit the severity of binges and diminish preoccupation with alcohol in abstinent alcoholics. Nausea has been a common side effect early in naltrexone treatment for alcoholism, but is generally mild and clears with continued use. Naltrexone can produce liver toxicity, which is dose dependent, has mainly been observed at much higher doses (200 or 300 mg per day), and resolves with dose reduction. Elevated liver enzymes, which do not resolve with dose reduction or discontinuation, represent another likely cause of hepatitis (e.g., viral, alcoholic).

Acamprosate has been approved for a number of years in Europe, and it recently received FDA approval. Its mechanism is not well understood but is thought to involve interference with excitatory amino acid mechanisms that may be involved in relapse. Clinical trials have shown a modest effect in reducing relapse risk, and studies are underway to determine if it may have complementary effects to those of naltrexone and whether the combination of the two may increase effectiveness. Acamprosate is supplied in 333 mg tablets, and the recommended dosage is two tablets, three times daily. Blister packs, organized according to the daily schedule of dosing, can be helpful to patients in maintaining compliance. Acamprosate is generally safe and well tolerated. Diarrhea is the most common side effect.

In the same way that any given antidepressant medication will be helpful to some depressed patients but not others, naltrexone and acamprosate may similarly have little effect in some patients but work well in others. As of yet, there are no reliable predictors of which alcohol-dependent patient will benefit from these medications, but clinicians should be encouraged to attempt adequate trials (effective dose, for at least a month) of these medications for patients with problem drinking, and not be discouraged by the fact that some patients will not benefit.

## Medications for Cocaine Dependence

Given the high relapse rates with psychosocial treatment alone, there has been considerable interest in the development of pharmacotherapies for cocaine dependence. Case reports and open pilot studies have suggested that a variety of agents may be effective but double-blind trials have provided disappointingly inconsistent results. Surveys have demonstrated that many addiction medicine specialists are using medicines to treat cocaine dependence despite the lack of evidence of a standard sufficient for FDA approval.

The most widely prescribed medicines for cocaine dependence are antidepressants. Depression occurs frequently in cocaine addicts and it is possible that antidepressants may correct neurotransmitter deficiencies associated with cocaine use. The best evidence relates to desipramine but early reports of its effectiveness in preventing relapse were subsequently contradicted and its efficacy for more than 6–12 weeks was questioned. Typical desipramine doses are the same as for the treatment of depression. Concurrent use of an antidepressant and cocaine increases the risk of additive cardiotoxicity and patients who recommence cocaine use during treatment should be assessed for this possibility.

Although antipsychotic drugs have been proposed on the grounds that blockade of dopamine receptors would attenuate the euphoric response to cocaine, experience treating patients with schizophrenia and cocaine dependence do not support this hypothesis. Furthermore, cocaine use is associated with dopamine depletion and may therefore increase the risk of extrapyramidal effects.

Psychomotor stimulants have been suggested as an agonist maintenance treatment strategy. Although early clinical reports suggested stimulants might exacerbate cocaine dependence, more recent placebo-controlled trials suggest oral dexedrine may have promise. Patients with attention deficit disorder, which commonly co-occurs with cocaine dependence, may benefit from stimulants. Similarly, the effectiveness of lithium in reducing cocaine use is confined to patients with comorbid bipolar disorder. The anticonvulsant carbamazepine had disappointing effects in controlled trials after initially promising results in open studies. However, more recently, some of the newer anticonvulsants with GABA-enhancing or excitatory amino acid inhibiting effects (e.g., topiramate, gabapentin) have shown promise in small placebo-controlled trials.

Interestingly, perhaps the most consistent data so far relate to disulfiram, which has shown promise in a series of small placebo-controlled trials for cocaine dependence, and the effect does not seem to depend on concurrent alcohol use. Since disulfiram inhibits dopamine a-hydroxylase, which catalyzes the conversion of dopamine to norepinephrine in the brain, it may promote increased levels of brain dopamine and combat the dopamine depletion engendered by cocaine.

Another pharmacotherapeutic strategy for cocaine dependence is to treat comorbid psychopathology, most commonly unipolar depression, bipolar disorder, attention deficit hyperactivity disorder, and anxiety disorders. Such treatment is most likely to have a direct impact on the psychopathology, followed by indirect effects of improved functioning and reduced drug use. The benefits of drug treatment in the absence of comorbid psychopathology is unclear. An effective pharmacotherapy for cocaine dependence is urgently needed.

## Medications for Opiate Dependence

Agonist maintenance treatment for opiate dependence is a powerful treatment with a large effect size. When properly prescribed, methadone will rapidly induce a dramatic remission in 50% or more of patients. It prevents or reduces illicit opiate use, craving for illicit opiates, criminal behavior associated with acquisition of illicit opiates, and diseases associated with illicit opiate use (such as illness related to infection with human immunodeficiency virus), and improves employment and other aspects of social functioning. Methadone has also been shown to reduce mortality rates among opioid dependent patients, in part by protecting against overdose. Methadone is also sometimes misunderstood as 'substituting one drug for another.' In fact, methadone works by inducing marked tolerance such that effects of other opiates are blocked, and no euphoric effects of the methadone itself are experienced. When prescribed with careful titration, methadone is neither intoxicating nor sedating, and it does not interfere with performance of functions that are important for responsible adult roles (e.g., studies have shown that methadone does not impair driving ability).

Methadone is well-suited for use as maintenance treatment. It is effective after oral administration and has a long half-life (>24 h); it suppresses opiate withdrawal syndrome for up to 36 h and it blocks euphoria induced by other opiates. Chronic administration is associated with minimal side effects, the most frequent of which are constipation, excess sweating, reduced sexual interest, but these rarely result in discontinuation of treatment.

The initial dose of methadone maintenance lies in the range 20–40 mg and this is mainly to relieve symptoms due to abstinence. This is followed by an 'induction period', in which the dose may be increased in increments of 5–10 mg until a dose is achieved that prevents opiate craving and blocks the euphoric effects of illicit opiates. Measures for patient monitoring include subjective reports, interval history, and regular frequent usine toxicology analysis. Although a dose of 40 mg/day may be sufficient for some patients, there is now evidence from several trials that most require 80 mg/day. According to Federal regulations, doses of methadone greater than 120 mg/day require permission, although individual states can specify lower ceiling doses. As with many psychopharmacologic treatments, the most common reason for treatment failure in methadone maintenance is inadequte dose, and continued opiate use should prompt consideration of a dosage increase. Some evidence suggests that optimal treatment response requires trough methadone blood levels in the range 200–400 ng/mL, and blood level monitoring may be useful in nonresponders. Some patients are rapid metabolizers, which can be assessed by comparing peak and trough blood levels. Rapid metabolizers may benefit from a divided, twice daily dose schedule.

A pragmatic drawback of methadone maintenance is that regulations stipulate that it can only be administered at specially licensed clinics that require frequent attendance (daily at the outset) and that are not even available in many geographic regions. This can be a practical constraint or a disincentive for many patients. On the other hand, it has been shown that the effectiveness of methadone maintenance depends upon regular counseling in conjunction with the medication, which is a requirement of methadone clinics, and more severely dysfunctional patients probably benefit from the structure imposed by clinic rules. Furthermore, many of the better methadone clinics offer primary medical and psychiatric care, which is important since chronic opiate-dependent patients often have multiple medical problems (e.g., hepatitis B and C, HIV) and psychiatric problems (e.g., depression, PTSD).

A recent development is the approval and marketing of the long-acting opiate partial agonist buprenorphine (see also the section above on opiate withdrawal on page 233), which has been shown in clinical trials to have effectiveness equivalent to that of methadone for maintenance treatment. A major difference is that buprenorphine can be prescribed by any physician who has taken a brief training course and received certification, making it more widely available than methadone maintenance. The main regulatory restriction is that individual physicians practicing in an office-based setting are restricted to treating no more than 30 patients with maintenance buprenorphine at any one time.

Buprenorphine has interesting pharmacologic properties. It is a partial agonist, meaning that it binds opiate receptors but only partially activates them. This may translate into lower abuse potential compared with full agonists, although buprenorphine has been abused by intravenous injections in other countries where it was widely available. The sublingual formulations marketed for treatment of opioid dependence do appear to have limited abuse potential by themselves, and the Suboxone formulation, which includes naloxone, discourages attempts to extract and inject the contents, since intravenous naloxone will precipitate withdrawal; the naloxone is poorly absorbed by the sublingual or oral routes. Buprenorphine binds almost irreversibly to opiate receptors, and dissociates very slowly, accounting in part for its long duration of action. When properly dosed, similarly to methadone, it induces tolerance, blocks the effects of other opiates, and produces little or no sedating or intoxicating effects.

The buprenorphine/naloxone combination (Suboxone) is preferred for both detoxification and maintenance treatment, although some patients may be more sensitive to the presence of the antagonist (naloxone) and tolerate straight buprenorphine (Subutex) better. Because it is a partial agonist, buprenorphine will precipitate withdrawal in individuals who have recently used any opioid drug; treatment should therefore begin when there are clear signs of withdrawal (or at least 4 h after last use of a short-acting opioid) (see also the section on buprenorphine for detoxification on page 234). There is less experience of induction with buprenorphine in individuals using long-acting agents such as methadone, but the risk of precipitated withdrawal is greater. The daily methadone dose should be below 40 mg per day before buprenorphine induction is attempted, and a delay of around 48 h or more is advisable to allow withdrawal symptoms from methadone to manifest clearly. Induction is completed over 2–4 days, depending on the target dose. The recommended dose on day 1 is 16 mg, increasing to 16 mg on day 2 and thereafter, and more gradual induction may be associated with a higher risk of drop-out. The dose should be adjusted in increments of 2–4 mg to that which keeps the individual in the treatment program and suppresses withdrawal symptoms; the target maintenance dose is 16 mg/day but may range from 4 to 32 mg/day. Buprenorphine should be administered as part of a psychosocial treatment program. The relative ease of withdrawing from buprenorphine may result in a greater tendency to leave the treatment program compared with methadone.

Owing to its long duration of action, buprenorphine can be administered every other day (e.g., 32 mg every other day), or even twice per week; this property can be useful for patients where there are concerns about compliance, since the medication can be held at a clinic or by a significant other and administered under observation on a less than daily basis.

Buprenorphine can produce sedation. However, emergence of sedation should also raise suspicion of use of other drugs or alcohol. Unlike full opiate agonists (heroin, methadone, other narcotic analgesics), where respiratory depression is a serious risk, buprenorphine by itself produces less respiratory depression. The rate of deaths from drug overdose dropped substantially in France after buprenorphine was introduced for treatment of drug dependence. The one exception was overdoses of buprenorphine in combination with benzodiazepines, where deaths were observed. This has led to an exaggerated concern that buprenorphine is contraindicated in patients who use benzodiazepines. For patients using benzodiazepines at regular, modest doses, which is the most common pattern even among opiate addicts, buprenorphine is safe. Patients who take large doses or binges of benzodiazepines are at risk of overdose in combination with a variety of other drugs, including buprenorphine, and alcohol. It is likely that the risk of overdose in such patients would be the same on either methadone maintenance or buprenorphine maintenance.

Naltrexone is a long-acting (24–48 h duration) opioid antagonist available in 50 mg tablets. It is effective in blocking the effects of opioids and can be used as a maintenance treatment, but its effectiveness has been limited by poor compliance. Compliance can be improved with behavioral therapy, but rates of retention in treatment still remain well below what can be expected from agonist maintenance with methadone or buprenorphine. Furthermore, naltrexone does not protect against opiate overdose; patients who stop naltrexone are not tolerant and are therefore vulnerable to overdose. Naltrexone is also complicated to manage. It cannot be started until a patient has been fully detoxified, in order not to precipitate withdrawal. Rapid induction methods using buprenorphine, clonidine, and clonazepam have been described, but generally require 5–7 days to carry out. Anesthesia-assisted rapid detoxification and induction onto naltrexone has been shown to involve the same level of discomfort, with increased risk of serious adverse events, and is not recommended. Once a patient is inducted onto naltrexone, if they stop taking the naltrexone and relapse, naltrexone cannot be resumed without precipitating withdrawal, and repeat detoxification is needed.

In summary, although some patients benefit from naltrexone, it is considered a second-line agent for patients who have failed or refuse agonist treatment. Patients maintained on naltrexone should be warned about the risk of fatal drug overdose if naltrexone is discontinued.

## Special Considerations

Two patient populations warrant particular comment: patients on medical-surgical units who are methadone-maintained and patients who are pregnant. When patients are admitted to hospital their maintenance program should be contacted to verify their methadone dose. This dose should be maintained, not reduced, during the stress of an illness and its treatment. Maintenance methadone will prevent opiate withdrawal but it will not provide analgesia. Patients who are in severe pain should therefore receive analgesia with a non-opiate or, bearing in mind that higher doses and shorter dose intervals may be needed, a short-acting opioid analgesic. Opioids with mixed agonist-antagonist properties, such as pentazocine and buprenorphine may precipitate withdrawal and should be avoided.

Longitudinal studies have shown that in utero exposure to methadone is not associated with abnormal development. Methadone maintenance should therefore be continued by women who become pregnant, though the dose may need to be reduced during the third trimester. The neonate may develop abstinence symptoms and this should be expected and treated after birth.

## Drug Treatments for Nicotine Dependence

Nicotine resembles other addictive drugs in that it induces similar addictive behavior patterns (such as inability to control consumption) and similar neuroadaptive changes (e.g., tolerance). Nicotine intoxication and withdrawal are not associated with the acutely harmful behavior that other drugs of abuse cause but the health consequences of nicotine make it the most important drug of abuse. Withdrawal symptoms associated with nicotine addiction include anxiety, restlessness, difficulty concentrating, and irritability. Drug treatment to prevent relapse in individuals with nicotine addiction must reduce these symptoms and in addition decrease craving for nicotine. This must be achieved in an environment with multiple conditional stimuli for nicotine use, such as the morning cup of coffee.

Nicotine can be delivered safely and its use gradually reduced using nicotine replacement therapy. By contrast with methadone maintenance, nicotine replacement therapy is not an indefinite maintenance treatment but it is worthwhile speculating whether nicotine replacement reduces harm compared with cigarette smoking. Nicotine replacement therapy is currently available as a transdermal patch and polacrilex 'gum' and both are effective in promoting abstinence.

The FDA recently approved a sustained-release formulation of bupropion for the treatment of nicotine dependence. It is as effective as nicotine replacement therapy. The suggested dose is 150 mg twice daily, beginnning two weeks before smoking cessation is attempted. In patients who derive no benefit from nicotine replacement or bupropion alone, a combination of the two therapies has been shown to be safe and more effective than monotherapy.

Many patients who succeed in initiating abstinence from cigarettes will relapse within 3–6 months. Clinicians and patients should not be discouraged by this. The data suggest that most patients who make repeated quit attempts eventually succeed in achieving sustained abstinence.

## PHARMACOTHERAPIES FOR SUBSTANCE ABUSERS WITH ADDITIONAL PSYCHIATRIC ILLNESS

There is consistent evidence that patients with psychiatric illness have higher than expected rates of substance abuse, and that patients undergoing treatment for substance dependence have higher than expected rates of psychiatric illness.

In this challenging patient population, clinical experience has confirmed that:

- treatment should be administered by health professionals with expertise in general psychiatry and chemical dependence
- it is unrealistic to insist on abstinence as a condition for treatment

- abstinence is not necessary for the safe and effective use of most psychotropic drugs
- symptom stability may be needed before a reduction in substance use is apparent
- substance use disorder tends to persist unless it is treated as an illness in itself, regardless of the effective management of other psychopathology

This section summarizes the management of particular psychiatric illnesses complicated by substance use and ends with a summary of important drug interactions in substance use disorders.

## Pharmacotherapy for Specific Psychiatric Disorders

It is difficult to be definitive about when a substance-induced mood disorder becomes a major depressive episode. According to most experts, there should be a period of sobriety lasting two weeks before a second diagnosis can be made in a patient presenting with a depressive syndrome. However, clinical trials have shown the benefit of antidepressant medication in patients who are not abstinent to begin with. Thus, there is room for clinical judgment, and, if significant depression persists and the patient cannot achieve abstinence, trials of antidepressant medications can be attempted. In a patient vulnerable to substance abuse relapse, the most worrying effects of antidepressant medication are cardiotoxicity (e.g., arrhythmias), neurotoxicity (e.g., seizures) or death from intentional overdose. These concerns are greatest with tricyclic antidepressants and the selective serotonin reuptake inhibitors have a safer pharmacologic profile. Although it is important to discourage individuals from using drugs of abuse, a significant number of people taking an antidepressant use alcohol and other potential drugs of abuse in moderation without ill effects. There seems to be little abuse potential with antidepressants though abuse of amitriptyline for its sedative effects and, more recently, fluoxetine for its stimulant effects, has been reported.

Substance abuse or dependence are frequent complications of schizophrenia; conversely, the psychotic symptoms that occur during drug intoxication and withdrawal complicate the diagnosis of schizophrenia. These patients need a particularly high degree of patience and sophisticated psychiatry services. Long-term follow-up (more than one year) of patients with schizophrenia and substance abuse suggests the need for energetic engagement in treatment for psychosis with an emphasis on compliance with antipsychotic medication and the maladaptive effects of substance misuse. The problem of substance abuse declines for most patients after a year of medication compliance and treatment for addiction. Long-acting depot antipsychotics are a rational component of such a strategy. A combination of medication and contingency contracting has also been used for patients with schizophrenia, in which unsupervised use of disability benefits is contingent on negative urine toxicology.

Substance-induced disorders (particularly stimulant intoxication and alcohol or sedative–hypnotic withdrawal) can resemble generalized anxiety disorder or panic attacks, and thus, as with depression, at least a two week period of abstinence is preferable prior to initiating pharmacotherapy, although again there is room for judgment. Other anxiety disorders, such as social phobia, agoraphobia, PTSD, or OCD, have distinctive symptoms that do not overlap with symptoms of toxicity or withdrawal. Behavioral approaches are effective for many anxiety disorders and should be considered, first alone and then as a supplement to pharmacotherapy. Antidepressants are effective for panic disorder or generalized anxiety disorder and have less abuse potential than the benzodiazepines. Buspirone may be beneficial for generalized anxiety disorder at a dose of at least 45 mg/day. If a benzodiazepine is still preferred, expert opinion (supported by some experimental evidence) suggests that the safest agents are oxazepam and chlordiazepoxide because their onset of action is more gradual and they have a lesser tendency to produce euphoria. In general, however, benzodiazepines should be avoided owing to their abuse potential.

Substance abuse and bipolar disorder (particularly in the manic phase) are frequently comorbid disorders but there is little information about the effects of treatments for bipolar disorder on substance abuse. Research in the treatment of alcohol and cocaine dependence suggests that concurrent use of lithium is relatively safe with regard to drug interactions but little is known about the risk of interactions between carbamazepine and valproate and drugs of abuse in patients with bipolar disorder.

Follow-up of children with attention deficit–hyperactivity disorder (ADHD) and conduct disorder has revealed high rates of substance abuse, and ADHD may be over-represented in substance abuse treatment settings. It is possible that patients with ADHD may seek stimulants for self-medication. The diagnosis of ADHD requires evidence of illness during childhood, preferably with verification from another person. These patients have benefited from methylphenidate, according to some reports. Desipramine and bupropion have been used successfully in treating children with ADHD and both have been advocated in patients with comorbid substance abuse.

## Drug Interactions in Chemical Dependency

Drug interactions in patients with chemical dependency may be pharmacodynamic or pharmacokinetic, and may occur between drugs of abuse or between drugs of abuse and prescribed medications.

### ALCOHOL

The combination of alcohol and cocaine has been associated with fatal cardiac events and increased hepatoxicity. Alcohol in combination with an opiate or cannabis cause greater sedation and greater neurologic impairment than when used alone. Acute alcohol intoxication is associated with inhibition of hepatic enzymes and may increase blood levels of concurrent medication. Conversely, chronic alcohol use causes enzyme induction, leading to lower blood levels of antipsychotic drugs, antidepressants, valproic acid, carbamazepine, and some benzodiazepines. Griseofulvin, metronidazole, chloramphenical and oral hypoglycemic agents may cause mild disulfiram-like reactions with alcohol. Alcohol and chloral hydrate compete for alcohol dehydrogenase; concurrent ingestion leads to higher blood levels of both and increased intoxication (this combination is known as a 'Mickey Finn').

## COCAINE AND OTHER STIMULANTS

The risk of tachycardia is greater with a combination of cocaine and cannabis than with either drug alone. A 'speedball' (heroin and cocaine) more easily produces respiratory depression than the single drugs. Taking cocaine or amphetamine during or shortly after treatment with a monoamine oxidase inhibitor can lead to hypertensive reactions.

## OPIATES

Methadone increases blood levels of concurrently taken antidepressants and zidovudine. Conversely, blood levels of methadone may be reduced to the point where abstinence symptoms occur by concurrent use of rifampin, phenytoin, barbiturates, and carbamazepine. The combination of meperidine and a monoamine oxidase inhibitor may cause extreme reactions ranging from collapse (hypotension and coma) to excitation (hypertension and convulsions).

## NICOTINE

Cigarette smoking reduces blood levels of caffeine; patients who stop smoking may therefore experience caffeine toxicity and this could be mistaken for nicotine withdrawal. Smoking also reduces blood levels of antipsychotic drugs, tricyclic antidepressants, theophyline, and propranolol.

## HALLUCINOGENS

A serotonin reuptake inhibitor reportedly exacerbated hallucinogen-persisting perception disorder (flashbacks) in adolescents with a history of LSD use. This is not surprising given the role of serotonergic mechanisms in hallucinogenic drug effects.

## ADDITIONAL READING

1. Substance Abuse: A Comprehensive Textbook (4th Edition). Edited by Lowinson JH, Ruiz P, Millman RB, Langrod JG. Lippincott Williams and Wilkins, Philadelphia, 2005
2. Principles of Addiction Medicine (3rd Edition). Edited by Graham AW, Schultz TK, Mayo-Smith MF, Ries RD, Wilford BB. American Society of Addiction Medicine, Inc., Chevy Chase, Maryland, 2003

3. Textbook of Substance Abuse Treatment (3rd Edition). Edited by Galanter M, Kleber HD. American Psychiatric Publishing, Inc., Washington, D.C., 2004

4. Clinical Textbook of Addictive Disorders (3rd Edition). Edited by Frances RJ, Miller SI, Mack AH. The Guilford Press, New York, 2005

5. International Handbook of Alcohol Dependence and Problems. Edited by Heather N, Peters T, Stockwell T. John Wiley and Sons Ltd., Chichester, UK, 2001

# INDEX

*Handbook of Psychiatric Drugs*  Jeffrey A. Lieberman and Allan Tasman
© 2006 John Wiley & Sons, Ltd

*Index prepared by Neil Manley*